BIGGER, FASTER, STRONGER

Better,

The World's Leading Fitness Experts Reveal Their

TOP SECRETS

To Help You

Achieve The Ultimate in

Health and Longevity

BIGGER, FASTER, STRONGER

Better,

The World's Leading Fitness Experts Reveal Their **TOP SECRETS** To Help You Achieve The Ultimate in Health and Longevity

Contents

CHAPTER 1

FIVE STEPS TO ACHIEVING ANY HEALTH AND FITNESS GOAL

By Sean Greeley

"Happiness lies, first of all, in health."
~ George William Curtis

To me, fitness is a way of life. Making (and keeping) a commitment to taking care of your health is critical to not only looking and feeling good, but giving your mind and body the strength it needs to reach your goals and be there for others who depend on you.

I enjoy pushing myself to work hard. My idea of relaxation is doing a Crossfit style workout until I'm nauseous. It doesn't sound like fun to many people, but, to me, achieving optimum fitness helps me to work and play at the highest level possible – and enjoy life to the fullest.

Fitness has also helped me to achieve many dreams - from being a top 400m runner in the New England Championships to being part of the USA Wakeboard team for three years and competing in both European and World Championships. I was also blessed to be able to successfully battle Stage IV cancer in 2003 and regain my complete health, to the point where I was recognized as one of the top personal trainers in the country by the American Council of Exercise in 2005.

At the same time, I've always admired systems. The right systems create success in whatever endeavor you might undertake – and it's helped me build a multi-million dollar business from the ground up. If there's a faster, easier and more profitable way to do something, I'll usually find it.

Since two of my big passions are systems and fitness, it was a natural next step to put them together to help people reap the benefits of good health as I have throughout my life. You may be one of the millions who are sick and tired of being... well, sick and tired. If so, this chapter will introduce you to my 5-step system – and give you the structure to begin turning around your health.

Let me share with you the 5 steps you can take to reach any fitness goal you have and live a better quality of life. These are the same 5 steps I've personally coached thousands of clients through when they make the commitment to feeling and looking better. Although I only have time to give you the broad strokes here, they will provide you with the basic blueprint to achieve your goals.

STEP ONE:
DEFINE YOUR GOALS, MOTIVATION AND COMMITMENT

Your mindset is all-important whenever you face any challenge – and improving your fitness is certainly no different. If anything, it's *more* important to be clear in your mind about what you want to achieve.

Start with your **goals**. If you're like most of the fitness clients I've worked with over the years, you're looking to reduce body fat, drop some weight, improve muscle tone and definition, increase your strength, and just develop a healthier lifestyle overall that leads to more energy and better vitality. But spend a few minutes getting more specific about those goals. Ask yourself these questions:

- If you want to lose weight, how much weight do you want to lose? If you want to build more muscle, how much muscle do you want to gain?

- If you want to improve your strength, by how much do you want to improve?

If you only have a more general goal, such as to just be healthier and feel better, that's fine – but a few specifics would help. This is the point when you should write down those specific goals – it may sound silly, but research shows that writing down goals, instead of just thinking or saying them, gives you more inner strength to achieve them.

Once you've written down those goals, think about WHY those goals are important to you. You must have a strong **motivation** to achieve them — understanding that motivation is key to moving forward.

For many folks that are new to fitness, they just want to improve their quality of life. Their weight has gradually gone up over the past few years, and the little things they've tried in the past to lose weight (like no longer drinking alcohol or cutting out the junk food) just aren't working anymore. They know it's time to do this thing right.

Other people are already in a program that just isn't giving them the results they want. Or they might have a special event coming up, like a wedding, a reunion, or a birthday party of note where they want to look their best.

Whatever your reason why, it has to be strong. So take time for some personal reflection and understand why you're doing this.

If you have your goals and your motivation worked out, you should now move on to your commitment. How committed are you to achiev ing your goals? Give yourself a personal ranking on a commitment scale from 1 to 10, with a "10" meaning you're willing to do "whatever it takes" to accomplish your goals.

Here's a little secret – if you view your commitment as anything less than that "10," you're not going to be very successful. So, whatever number you assigned to your commitment, ask yourself why you chose it.

Many people give themselves lower scores because they struggle with knowing what to do to be successful. Maybe they don't know how to exercise appointments. This is where a coach or trainer can really be of use – they hold you accountable, give you the knowledge you need to make a program work, and provide the support to lead you through to success.

STEP TWO:
PERFORM AN INITIAL EVALUATION

This is where you find your starting point. It's important to know where you began so you can measure your progress along the way. You can have a trainer help you with this, or perform a simple Fitness Assessment on your own. Either way the assessment should include measuring the things you seek to change. For example:

- Weighing yourself on a scale
- Taking some measurements of your body
- Taking a body fat assessment (which many scales now offer today as a built-in calculation)
- Completing a profile of your current nutrition habits
- Taking some "before" photographs of your body

Now, let me say that I don't know *anyone* who enjoys doing an assessment of their body, particularly when they're already unhappy about where they are. But try to get past that and do it anyway.

The photos may be the hardest part. While nobody likes to look at a less-than-desirable photograph of themselves, some initial "before" photos will provide you with a great reference in the future for those times when you say, "I don't feel like anything's happening." Comparing a photograph of yourself every three to six weeks will allow you to *really start seeing changes occur* and *you'll get excited about the results*. That way you'll be more motivated to continue with your program and do everything-it-takes to be successful in achieving your goals.

STEP THREE:
DESIGN YOUR PROGRAM

Steps 1 and 2 helped you decide where you want to go and locked down where you're starting from. Now it's time to connect the dots and plot your course. You need to create a road map to get you from where you are now to where you want to be.

This may be a little difficult to do on your own, as it requires a wide knowledge of fitness and nutrition. Let me share with you what I call the "The Six Proven Components of Success."

1. **Nutrition** - the foundation of all health and fitness

2. **Supplementation** - to fill in the voids in your nutrition program

3. **Resistance training** - to build lean muscle and ramp up the metabolism

4. **Cardiovascular exercise** - to optimize fat burning and heart health

5. **Flexibility** - to prevent injury and promote recovery from exercise

6. **Coaching** - knowledge, support and accountability to get you to the finish line

1. We'll start with #1 –**nutrition.** Nutrition is the foundation of all health and fitness. I work with my clients to create meal plans and make a grocery list of the foods that are helpful. You should have an *exact plan of what you need to eat* in a day to be successful – and then simply check off those items as you go through your day. If the plan is solid and you follow it, you're going to see results.

2. Once you start eating better, you'll find that your energy will increase and your metabolism will start working again. You also, however, need to address the second component, **supplementation,** to fill in the voids in your diet and provide your body with the nutrients you're not getting from your food.

There are three main supplements I recommend to all of my clients. Number one is a good multi-vitamin/mineral supplement. Why? Because every major medical and health organization in America today now recommends you take a multi-vitamin or multi-mineral supplement for complete nutrition. In addition to a good multi-vitamin/mineral supplement, we also recommend additional anti-oxidants like vitamin C, vitamin E, an additional B-complex and, unless you're eating a ton of red meat, additional iron.

I also recommend using a meal replacement product to all of my clients because I don't know anyone who can realistically eat a complete meal six times a day and have a normal life. That's why having the convenience of a good, balanced meal-replacement shake or bar is great in between your major meals, or even for breakfast-on-the-go.

Third, I recommend having a post-workout recovery shake. After your resistance training or strength training workout, a recovery shake is critical to transferring your muscles into the recovery phase. Putting your body into the recovery phase fast allows you to reduce muscle soreness and start rebuilding and repairing tissue right away. That way you can maximize the effort you put in at the gym and get the best results from your workout in the shortest period of time.

3. Let's look at our third "Component of Success" – **resistance training,** the first part of our exercise regimen.

Your resistance training program should be designed to build lean muscle, get your metabolism going, and increase your strength. I recommend a combination of functional-type and weight-type training exercises. That way, you're challenging your body completely - not just the big muscles, but also the little ones, so they can actually support your body, the way you move in the real world.

4. Now, let's move on to **cardiovascular exercise.** You want to focus on this for heart health and to optimize your body's ability to burn fat 24/7. As a general rule, for good health and weight management, everyone should aim for at least three non-consecutive days of cardiovascular activity each week. Traditional cardio includes running outdoors or on a treadmill, elliptical machines, rowers, regular or stationary bikes, aerobic classes, stairsteppers, etc. Swimming, rollerblading outside, mountain biking, and cycling are all great outdoor cardio activities. But for efficiency and time effectiveness, I would encourage you to focus on INTERVAL training for your cardiovascular exercise. You can also mix up your resistance training to include intervals for a power-packed punch of intensity and efficiency.

5. Our next component is **flexibility.** You need to prepare your body for a workout every day to prevent injury, promote the recovery process and just get your body moving better again – and you need to cool down afterwards.

A good warm-up should last anywhere from 5 to 10 minutes and should include some low-intensity cardiovascular exercise, like walking on the treadmill, jogging, biking or some cardio-calisthenics. This will prepare you to then spend another 5-10 minutes per- forming the warm-up stretching exercises, get in tune with your body that day, and get ready to have a great workout.

Likewise, after you've done the workout, it's a MUST that you spend time cooling down. Doing so allows you to flush out lactic acid, toxins, and other waste products that are left over in your muscles from exercise. Flushing these toxins out with some light cardiovascular exercise and stretching again will reduce delayed onset muscle soreness (that feeling like you can't walk for several days), and (along with post-workout nutrition) will accelerate your body's recovery process. The cool down should also be around 5 to 10 minutes or so.

6. The final component is **coaching.** My job as a coach is to provide my clients with the knowledge to create a good program and eliminate the "guesswork" for you. My expertise comes from years of study and working hands-on in the trenches coaching my clients. I already know what works and what doesn't. You need a coach with the same level of experience who can support you through your program.

STEP FOUR:
PUTTING YOUR PROGRAM INTO ACTION

Once we review our clients' plans, we make it their next step to start taking the action they need to take, in order to get the results they want. It's time to get off the bench and get in the game – and that means you have to learn the components of the program, and you have to learn new habits.

Here's a newsflash: You already have fitness and nutrition habits in your lifestyle right now; they're just habits that aren't getting you to where you want to get. It's time to change those habits out for better ones.

The first 3 weeks of program implementation are critical. Studies show that it takes around 21 days to integrate a new habit into your life. Think about it—you don't have to consciously tell yourself to brush your teeth in the morning, take a shower or get that cup of coffee when you wake up it's just part of your routine every day.

Similarly, you want to build good habits around exercise and nutrition so you can maintain your results and always be where you want to be. If you follow this plan for 21 days, you're going to have to think about it at first to get things going. But, once you get on track, it becomes automatic. You'll be on auto pilot with your new habits and your success will be guaranteed.

STEP FIVE:
REGULARLY ASSESS YOUR RESULTS
& UPDATE YOUR PROGRAM

As you progress through your program, regularly evaluate your progress and results. Doing so will allow you to gauge where you are on your "road map," make any course corrections that are necessary, and continue to your destination. I recommend you mark on your calendar the dates (about every 3 weeks) for you to update your evaluation. Measure everything just like you did the first day of your program.

It's been proven time and time again that people always perform better, whether it's in their job or in sports, when their results are measured. That's why runners are timed, why accountants prepare monthly P/L statements, and why we keep score in football. Measuring your activity and results is an absolute must. You MUST evaluate yourself at regular intervals throughout this program. That way you can hold yourself accountable for your results, prevent any backsliding, and stay on track with your plan to achieve your goals.

Again, this chapter featured the broad strokes of the system I've shared over the years with all our clients – many of the subjects we covered here could (and should) have their own chapter. In fact, these are the exact same steps I use with other business owners today to help them grow their fitness business. The steps work to improve anything you desire... not just your health and fitness. If you visit my website at: www.FitnessMarketingMuscle.com, you'll see many testimonials as well as real "before" and "after" pictures of my clients (today they are testimonials related to business success instead of fitness results). They're serious proof that I've gotten tremendous success stories from this program in working with my clients.

Everyone deserves a long life filled with health and happiness. Taking the right approach to fitness and nutrition helps you achieve that goal. I wish you luck in achieving all your goals and living your life to the fullest.

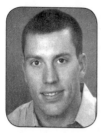

ABOUT SEAN

Sean is all about making the most from all you've got. As a professional Wake Boarder he rose to the very highest level, representing team USA at the World Championships in Germany. As a Fitness business owner, again he far surpassed what many of his peers in the industry dreamed of accomplishing, creating a 653-strong client base in just 3 years, starting from nothing. Sean was also recognized as one of the Top 10 Personal Trainers in the country.

Now with NPE, Sean (along with Eric) has started a business from scratch and turned it into a multi-million dollar, industry-leading company in just two years. This feat was recognized by the very best business builders in the world at the Glazer Kennedy Info-Summit 2008 where Sean & Eric won the "Info Marketers of the Year" award.

Sean's biggest asset is his ability to systemize and then maximize almost every business essential — from sales, to marketing, to management and more. If there's a faster, easier and more profitable way to do something, Sean will find it.

In his spare time, Sean likes to "relax" by cranking out nausea-inducing Cross-Fit workouts, surfing in oftentimes shark-infested waters, or being pulled at up to 23mph, hanging onto the back of a wakeboarding boat.

CHAPTER 2

Your **ENERGY STAR** Metabolism

By Chris & Jessica Page

A few years back we came home from a short trip only to find our cheap, low-end refrigerator had kicked the bucket while we was gone. We purchased the lower quality model to save a couple of hundred bucks, against the salesman's advice I might add. We knew we were taking a risk, but didn't see the value in spending the extra money. The irony of the old saying, "don't say I didn't warn you" really hit home, especially while we were in the middle of throwing away warm, thawed meat, spoiled milk and rotten eggs without the protection of a chemical warfare suit. We had learned our lesson from this and were bound and determined to make a higher-quality purchase the second time around.

Just like a potential training client probes for answers on what services we offer, what our success rates are, how we're going to go about helping them reach their goals and what the cost will be, we probed our salesman on similar points; how is the product ranked with Consumer Reports, what is the warranty, how much energy will it use and what's the price? Of course, this experience taught us that we get what we pay for, so we purchased a product with an excellent rating from Consumer reports and one that was Energy Star efficient. This is when it all started to hit home.

This experience preempted a snowball effect that forever changed the way we work with our clients. Now I'm sure you're wondering how these two things can possibly have anything remotely in common.

Let's compare. Our first refrigerator was cheaply made, barely did it's job and wasn't at all energy efficient. The new refrigerator is high quality, always keeps our food cold and uses a lot less energy to do it. What we really wanted from the first refrigerator wasn't at all what we ultimately purchased. We wanted a quality product that did what it was supposed to do and peace of mind that it would do it without fail, but ultimately purchased the opposite. This is similar to the client who wants results but ultimately purchases a gym membership instead of the expertise of a professional trainer.

Again, what does all of this have to do with fitness and exercise? An ENERGY STAR refrigerator and the efficiency of the human body have some similarities. Before we can elaborate, we need to go back in time to understanding how our own energy efficiency developed. The human body is designed for survival. Ten thousand years ago there were no supermarkets and gourmet restaurants. We had to hunt our food, chase our food, and kill it in order to eat. This meant we became very good at running. Unfortunately, meals would be few and far in between. Since our bodies didn't know when we'd feed it again, our metabolisms slowed to a grinding halt in order to reserve fat for energy. Our bodies evolved to being very efficient at storing fat, as fat is our survival fuel. Basically we became our own energy star appliance, burning a lot less energy or calories to keep us alive, essentially slowing our metabolisms to reserve fat for the long durations between meals – what we call starvation or famine mode. This is why you always hear health and fitness experts telling you to eat four or five small meals a day. If you constantly feed your body nutrient-dense foods, in the right ratios and quantities, your metabolism will run higher to burn the excess calories. You're basically tricking your body into thinking there is no famine to contend with. This is why it's better to eat five small meals of four hundred calories than two large meals of one thousand calories. Although both scenarios' consist of two thousand calories, how our body responds to the duration in between these meals makes all the difference between revving your metabolism and burning calories or slowing it and storing calories.

Now that you have a very basic understanding of the physiological history behind our metabolism, let's talk movement. The human body was meant to run. It's how we did our shopping back then. The better, or more efficient, we became at that movement, the less calories we'd burn doing it – that's conservation of energy and another big benefit toward our survival. Today, you would be hard pressed to drive through any town, at any time of day, and not see at least one walker or runner, if not a group of walkers and runners. But is this our best choice for movement? This is where our Energy Star Principle comes from; the more efficient you are at any movement, the less energy output you'll have doing a movement.

If you're just starting an exercise program that consists of walking, you should be applauded. Anything you do to get started on an exercise program is better than parking your butt on the couch. Just remember, we are designed to do this type of movement, which means sooner rather than later you'll be very efficient at walking and you'll need a greater stimulus, such as running – in order to generate a substantially greater caloric burn. At some point, you'll want to re-evaluate what the biggest bang for your buck really is. For example, let's say the average newbie to a walking program moves at a blistering 2.5 mph and they walk for an hour. The average person will burn approximately 80-100 calories for every mile per hour that they walk. So in this scenario you'd burn a maximum of 250 calories in an hour. If you walked five days a week, it would take almost three weeks to burn one pound of body fat (3500 calories per pound of fat divided by 1250 calories burned in a week). This is where intensity comes into play. If you increase your speed to a 5 mph jog you would double the number of calories burned in an hour and lose that pound of body fat twice as quick. Still though, not great numbers being put up on the score board. And, we're a far cry from a well-rounded exercise program.

If you really don't want an energy star body and you don't, then you can't be a couch potato in the gym either. What I'm talking about here is getting your butt off the machines. Machine circuits are the nightmare professional strength coaches and personal trainers of the world can't wake up from. Every client wants to know how to work the machines. Visit any franchise gym and you'll find plenty of machines in use. Mike Boyle once said something to the effect of, "look and see what everyone around you in the gym is doing and then do the opposite." That's exactly how we feel about machine circuits. There is nothing functional about a machine. Machines don't stimulate our core musculature or our neuro-muscular patterns, they certainly can't improve balance awareness, you won't burn any significant number of calories exercising on a machine, and you will never be a better athlete. You are an athlete by the way. You probably won't be body-checking or tackling anyone anytime soon, but life is a game of survival. Tripping, slipping and falling are an unfortunate part of life. You don't need to study the theories of Sir Isaac Newton to believe in gravity. One good fall and you'll know gravity exists. And all the intense training you've given your butt from sitting on a machine won't help you because your balance and coordination will be suppressed.

Another pitfall to working on machines is that it's generally easy. You take a seat on the machine, catch your breath, push a pin in the desired weight position, and move the weight in a restricted range of motion that isolates a group of muscles. When you're done, you sit and relax contemplating on where you're going for lunch. When the time is right, you do it again before moving to the next machine with great focus and intensity. Now don't get us wrong, this isn't a completely terrible plan if you're totally new to fitness or have some physical challenges. It's better to do something over nothing, right? Maybe! But the majority of the adult population has a job that has us sitting for long periods of time throughout the workday. Does it really make any sense to sit down to exercise?

To throw another wrench in the fitness wheel, humans are creatures of habit and comfort. Habits, good or bad, can be created in three weeks. Once you get into this routine, it becomes comfortable and this is where the bigger problems lie. First, it only takes about two weeks and then your body starts to become complacent to the stimulus that you're giving it and efficient to the movement. If you're a regular to fitness, then you've most likely heard of the Plateau Effect. As described by Wikipedia, a plateau effect occurs when a formerly effective measure ceases to cause further change. The tasks at hand become easier to perform and therefore you are more efficient at doing it. Second, comfortable usually means low intensity and you saw how simply going from a walk to a jog affected calorie burning.

If you really do want the benefits associated with exercise then you need to come out of your comfort zone. You will never attain any substantial fitness goals doing fuzzy-wuzzy, feel-good fitness on a machine. You will not substantially increase your metabolism and strength or decrease body fat. You will not improve motor skills, balance, coordination, or core strength. You certainly can't improve functional strength which is really the most important kind. You will however have an Energy Star metabolism that's good at storing fat and bad at burning calories.

So exactly how did this experience forever change the way we work with our clients? As you can probably guess, we don't sit them on a machine to get work done. Almost every bit of scientific research tells us that the best way to train is through functional training and dynamic movements. This doesn't mean standing one-legged on a BOSU® ball while doing bicep curls with 10 pound dumbbells. If your workout routine involves similar versions and appears acrobatic in nature, then it's time to re-evaluate. It's these kinds of workouts, commonly found in fitness magazines, which are turning gyms into circus shows. These types of activities are not considered to be functional training exercises and rarely improve strength, although they may help your balance. Functional refers to training specific movement patterns such as pushing, pulling, flexing (or bending) and extending - without losing the strength component. Cross-Training is a great way to increase your metabolism, strength and power, while blasting fat. This type of training uses different forms of exercise to train the entire body, not just target specific muscle groups like machines. This produces an overall higher level of all-around conditioning and reduces the risk of injury. You're also less likely to get bored, and you will definitely be working outside your exercise comfort zone.

Energy Star Efficiency and the Plateau Effect are two really good reasons to come out of your comfort zone, get off the machines and increase your workout intensity. We run a functional, cross-training boot camp at our facility that incorporates many different variations of the following functional strength movements: pushing and pulling, sled work, deadlifts and squats, along with core exercises like anti-rotation. We incorporate conditioning activities such as battling ropes, biking, calisthenics, plyometrics, and agility work. And we throw in some upper and lower body power activities such as power push-ups and box jumps. To round everything out, there's always mobility and flexibility work done, especially for the hip flexors. These types of workouts are fun, they burn an enormous amount of calories, usually 800-1200 in an hour, and they keep your body from getting stale.

Here's the gist of keeping your body from becoming Energy Star efficient:

- First, eat more often, not less. If your diet requires two thousand calories a day then break this up into five meals of four hundred calories each.

- Second, increase your work intensity to substantially burn more calories in the same amount of time.

- Third, get off the machines. Sitting down to get fit is an oxymoron. This is a big deal if you're serious about improving your fitness level.

- That leads us to number four, get functional. Functional training is the best type of training you can do. It's how all professional athletes train and so should you. What we mean by this is to do exercises that have you driving the ground, engaging your core musculature, developing nervous system/muscular system coordination, and do it under an appropriate resistance that improves strength.

- Fifth, watch what you read in magazines. Although some have great ideas to shake up your routine, these workouts are never a one-size-fits-all solution. Do your own evaluation of the exercises described in articles to be sure they're the right stimulus for your metabolism.

- Finally, don't be afraid to ask a professional for help. You already use different types of professionals every day to guide you in the right direction: Your physician evaluates and treats an injury or illness; your financial advisor guides you towards smart investments; your lawyer protects you from legal threats; and your accountant from financial doom. Just like these specialists, your professional trainer is there to help you safely reach your fitness goals through proper exercise prescription.

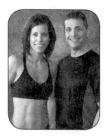

ABOUT CHRISTOPHER & JESSICA

Christopher and Jessica Page are co-owners of Page Fitness Athletic Club, a professional training facility in Watertown, New York. Together they built a team of professional trainers and fitness experts who are some of the most highly sought after and foremost experts in their field, and are regularly featured in the media.

Chris served in the United States Air Force from 1989 - 1994 during which he was a student of the Shou Shu martial art and veteran of the Persian Gulf War. In 1998 he graduated from the University of Kentucky with a Bachelor's Degree in Exercise Science and became certified as a Strength Coach through the National Strength & Conditioning Association. Chris has trained hundreds of athletes ranging from Junior High School through Semi-Professional status – including Army Rangers, Special Forces, Police, DEA and FBI agents.

Jessica is a Licensed Massage Therapist who began teaching group fitness in 2005. In 2009, she became a LesMills International, certified BODYPUMP™ instructor and Certified with Distinction in BODYCOMBAT™. Jessica has an enormous passion for fitness, which led her to compete in the Fitness America Pageants. In 2009, she won the Model Capitol Championships in Annandale, Virginia and was a Top 10 finalist in the International Fitness America Pageant in Miami, Florida.

Today, they have founded what has now become the number one training facility in Northern New York, and offer an unprecedented, 100% money-back guarantee on their training services. To receive a Free Fitness Consultation or to learn more about the training and health services their facility offers, visit: www.PageFitness.com or call the facility direct at (315) 786-8032.

CHAPTER 3

Six Rules For A Healthy, Happy, And More Fulfilling Life

By J.R. Kuchta

My journey into health and fitness began back in high school. I was athletic and had great speed, but to quote the janitor in the movie Rudy, "I was 5 foot nothing, one hundred and nothing." My diminutive stature led me to the weight room to try to improve the only thing that was in my control, my strength. This was Lincoln, Nebraska in 1995, no Internet and no strength and conditioning coach. Sure we had "Weight Training" class, but this consisted of running a couple of laps and then being put in a weight room while our teacher, the head football coach, sat in his office drawing up plays. Looks like I was on my own. So where did I turn? Fitness magazines.

The guys on the cover of the magazines were monsters, so obviously they must be following the routines and taking the supplements listed inside. I needed to look like this... NOW! So to get stronger I started do body building routines. Whoops.

Well, fast forward 17 years and take a look on any magazine rack. Unless you are at a mega bookstore, I can guarantee that you won't find a single magazine that is dedicated solely to strength, flexibility, and health maintenance. And why is that? Because unless the workout is going to give you 20 inch biceps, ripped six-pack abs, or a tight tush, people don't want it.

Needless to say, my fitness journey has been a long and circuitous one, and really it is still in its infancy. I'm 33 years old and most would consider me an expert in my field. After studying Exercise Science and obtaining several certifications, I find that the more knowledge I gain, the more I realize how much I *don't* know. And while on some level this is frustrating, on another it is very exciting. There is still so much that is unknown about exercise, nutrition, and performance. Everyday new information is coming out, and along with that are new methods to improve people's lives. There are so many variables to a person's performance: the workouts performed, weights used, rest periods, hormone levels, nutritional profiles and on and on.

So, if I am still seeking answers, I can only imagine what someone with very little health and fitness knowledge is going through. Most people struggle when they attempt to get fit and healthy because they pick up the fitness magazines and want to look like the cover model. For females, it is the tall, slender physique, with the ultra narrow waist. For guys it is the never-ending quest for sculpted pecs, swollen biceps, and six-pack abs. Our ideal body image is unrealistic and for 99% of the population, unattainable and unhealthy. These cover models not only have great genetics, but most use drugs and severe, restrictive dieting to achieve their physiques.

And once you set this image as your ideal, you are absolutely doomed. I left bodybuilding behind years ago, but still buried inside me is that 16-year-old kid wanting to be big and ripped. Every once in a while he'll pop out and I'll have to smack him back into place. The psychology behind your body image is powerful – and very, very difficult to change.

Then throw a certain popular weight-loss show into the mix and now people are doubly doomed. Because you see it on TV, you want and expect to lose 8, 10, 15 lbs in one week! What you might not realize is that you'd be comparing your fitness and weight loss results to people who have NO jobs, several HOURS of training a day, and a chef cooking their meals for them. I blame this show for many of my clients being *disappointed* with losing 3 lbs in a week.

I don't mean to just bash fitness magazines and weight loss TV shows. Very often, you *can* find good information buried inside the fitness magazines. And although I am often appalled at what I see on TV, many of the contestants' stories *are* inspiring and I find the training sessions interesting to watch. Fitness magazines and "reality" weight loss TV shows shape the ideas of what most people see as health and fitness though, and for that I am worried.

If you find that most of your ideas about health and fitness have been shaped by magazines and TV, I want to make a difficult appeal to you. One that, if followed, will profoundly change not just your body, but also your mind and self-image. Chances are that you aren't happy with your body and current state of health. You want to be thinner and more healthy, right? You've tried diets, you've tried exercise and still you struggle. Why? Because you are desperately trying to change what you see in the mirror first. You are "pushing" fitness and nutrition (dieting) on yourself as a means to burn calories and get rid of fat.

My appeal to you is to take just 3 months and choose performance over appearance. Concentrate on fitness and nutrition as an end in itself, not just as the means to a thinner body. Focus on getting stronger, more flexible, faster, developing more endurance, and choosing more nutrient dense foods. When you use fitness and food in this manner you will end up "pulling" the desired body composition results you desire. If you can follow the 5 rules that I outline below for just 3 months, I can guarantee a healthier, happier, more fulfilling life.

1. Train like an athlete.

You may not be interested in competition and may not consider yourself an athlete, but you should definitely train like one. Training like an athlete will help you to achieve more balance, flexibility, and strength. It will force you to work on your weaknesses and constantly strive for better performance.

This means you should ditch the endless row of machines at the gym and wander over to the small section of the gym where the dumbbells and barbells are. Most of the machines put our bodies in unnatural positions and require a single joint to do the exercise. The only machine you should be using is your body! In real life movement when are we ever required to simply move just one joint? Very, very, rarely, …if ever. Shoveling snow? Doing laundry? Getting out of your chair? All multi-joint movements. So TRAIN using multi-joint movements. Squats, deadlifts, presses, pull ups. All of these exercises prepare and train your entire body, while also working balance and flexibility.

2. Select premium fuel for your body.
Sadly, many people care more about the gas they put in their car than the food they put in their mouths. If you own a luxury sedan and it says to put premium fuel in the vehicle, do you just shrug your shoulders and pump in the cheap stuff? No, you grit your teeth and give your car premium.

You are a luxury sedan and deserve premium fuel too! But most people are choosing the cheap stuff. Fast food and processed foods are killing us. What's worse is we know it, and aren't doing anything about it. But not you. You are going to choose premium foods. Your primary food choices should be garden vegetables, lean meats, some fruits, and very little nuts and oils. I want you to limit your starches and eliminate sugar and grains. Fat isn't making you fat; sugar and grains are making you fat. If you only followed one piece of my advice, please make it be to swear off sugar and greatly limit grains. Your body and your kids and grandkids will thank you. Your body will thank you because you will feel, perform, and look much better. Your kids and grandkids will thank you because you will actually be around for them and not die off due to the host of lifestyle diseases that sugar can contribute to: obesity, diabetes, and cardio-vascular disease to name a few.

3. Work on your self-image – this is a constant effort.

We are human beings and even the most confident and positive people have moments, situations, and time periods of self-doubt and negativity. The harder you work on building a positive self image, the thicker your armor will be to the onslaught of negative forces, people, and messages that we are bombarded with. Read positive, reinforcing self-help books that build you up and get you motivated. Sit down, think hard, and actually write down the negative views you have about yourself and work on them. If you have negative self-worth, you will get poor results in whatever you attempt to achieve; so fix this, now.

4. Find a GOOD Coach.

You are fully capable of learning food and nutrition concepts on your own, but your progress will be greatly accelerated by a coach. There is so much misinformation out there, that a good coach will cut through the rubbish and shine a light on the good information. A coach is there for the good times and the bad times. They can keep you accountable and they don't let you rationalize and make excuses for yourself. A coach motivates and encourages you. Most importantly, a good coach will make sure you are doing exercises properly, eating the right things at the right times, and challenging yourself.

5. Spend as much on your health and fitness as you do on your car payment.

This is no joke. Most of us spend 200, 300, even 500 dollars a month for the car we drive, but can't shell out $50 a month for a gym membership? Come on, wake up! When you look back at your life, are you going to wish "Man, I really should have up-graded to the CLS package that had the larger alloy wheels and nicer wood-grained trim..." No, you will not. You are going to be looking up at your family and wished, "Man, I really should have taken care of myself. I'm not going to see my daughter get married and I'm not gonna be there to watch and help raise my grandchildren."

When you leave this world, leave an image of health, well-being, and vitality. Don't spend the last 20 years of your life in decline, complaining, and having your kids arguing over who has to take care of you. Decisions you make right now can and will impact far more than just yourself. If you don't do it for yourself, do it for your family.

6. Incorporate 'fun' & 'different' into your workout routine.
You shouldn't be doing the same mundane workout over and over again. 20 minutes on the treadmill, 20 minutes of weight training using the endless circuit of machines... YAWN. Repeat. Your body quickly adapts to any routine and after an initial period of rapid improvement, results will come to a screeching halt. Continue to seek out new, fun things to do to supplement your exercise and keep it fresh and engaging. Try out a new skill such as Tae Kwon Do, or even Swing Dancing. It will provide a new stimulus to both your mind and your muscles. By continuing to add new learning stimuli, your brain has to continue to create new neural pathways to accomplish these tasks. This can result in a smarter, sharper you as you age.

So there you have it. By following the **Six Rules** outlined above and NOT concentrating on the number you see on the scale, you are going to see dramatic, life-changing improvements. If you think I am wrong, just try it for three months and I will prove it to you.

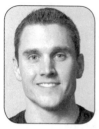

About JR

J.R. Kuchta is a health and fitness expert that is constantly searching for new and more practical ways to help improve people's lives. In 2007, J.R. ditched a successful corporate finance career to follow his passion for health and fitness and he has not looked back since. First, he obtained the Certified Personal Trainer designation from the International Sports Sciences Association. Then, his quest for more knowledge and fitness information led him to acquire a CrossFit Level 1 Trainer certification from CrossFit. Now he is studying under one of America's leading fitness and health pioneers, James Fitzgerald, to obtain the designation of Optimum Performance Training Master Coach.

Benefiting from J.R.'s health and fitness explorations have been the clients at Solution 1 Fitness, his personal training business, located in Johnson County, Kansas. Along with a staff of top-notch trainers, J.R. has helped hundreds of clients achieve new levels of health, fitness, and overall happiness through fitness training and nutritional coaching.

You won't find 'cookie cutter' workouts or run-of-the-mill nutrition advice at Solution 1 Fitness, either. J.R. believes that the current information on health, fitness, and nutrition is extremely cluttered with misinformation, outdated advice, myths, and downright lies. His passion is directed at constantly researching and experimenting with better ways to train and eat, not only for short-term performance, but also for long-term health and quality of life.

Get all the latest health and nutrition info by visiting J.R.'s website at: www.solution1fitness.com.

CHAPTER 4

The Achiever's Mindset

By Rick Martinez

Hi there. My name is Rick and my career has been as a health care provider – a registered nurse actually. Most of my years were in a variety of emergency departments around the U.S. and a stint in the US Army as an Army nurse. And kind of a key point, I think, is that I was a fat kid growing up and a chubby adult into my early 30's. Until a few short years ago that is. It was 12 minutes that changed my life… resolved my mind and it is exactly those 12 minutes that I focus on each and every time I am faced with a client that says "can't"…or asks "why"… or yes, even cries. I'd like to share with you what it was that changed my life forever, and subsequently catapulted our fitness organization into the "Best of the City" in San Antonio, Texas, and soon got us recognized as the best coaches around.

But it's not about us…this is about you. …And your winning *mindset*.

THE STORY

The power of the mind. We've all heard stories or seen movies about it. There's the movie "Rudy"…about the kid who just won't give up. There's Steve Prefontaine…an iconic runner who overcame adversity just by sheer will alone. Then there's even Ali… "fly-like-a-butterfly" Ali who seemed to beat his opponents before even stepping into the ring. They had a *mindset* that said nothing would stop them. Ever.

But we're here to talk about fitness. Fitness…wellness…health and beauty….looking better naked…it's all essentially the same thing, but the paths we individually choose to achieve those goals are what makes a program a program. Even more so is the *mindset* going into a program and understanding that fitness and wellness is a life-long journey.

And it begins with the right *mindset*. The desire to want to achieve.

It's a very easy word to write…"mindset"…and a very easy word to say, "Yup, I got this"…but do we? Do you? And how do you know?

Allow me to share a story about *mindset*, and what I believe really is a state we each individually must arrive at to accomplish any goal we set out to. In 2006 I was an Army nurse at Walter Reed Army Medical Center. I was working on a ward famous because our patients were amputees. Young men and women who had recently lost something in service to country. I bet you think this story is about a young hero who lost a leg, and became determined to run again. Right?

Wrong.

This story is about his mom. I had been a registered nurse for well over a decade by this time. It was 5:45 am on my first day at Walter Reed. My very first day. I walked into the report room, flipped on the lights and quickly realized there was a young lady asleep in the room…on the couch. She was all of 5'1", I would say about 35 years old, brown eyes and dark hair, very average looking. She stood up and folded her hospital blanket, which I am sure the night nurse had offered her to use. Hospitals, you know, can be a cold place. She placed the blanket, very nicely folded by now, on top of her plastic hospital pillow and set them both down, very meticulously, on the edge of the couch she had just gotten up from. She kind of straightened out her shirt with her hands…ran her hands down her pant legs to smooth them out…as best she could. Fixed her collar. She moseyed over to the sink with her overnight bag. I watched her…kind of curiously. I said "good morning" and watched as she made her way to the sink with her hand towel and make-up bag. She paused a second and just looked at herself in the mirror. I was just aimlessly watching her…not sure what was going on. I was in uniform. My ACU's. Fresh haircut. Even today the aftershave I used still fills my nostrils as I think about this. Vivid.

The pause, now that I think about it, was more than a pause. It was a reflection and though it's hard to describe in a book chapter…I really believe she was looking *through* her eyes in the mirror. I really believe she wasn't seeing her reflection, but looking really deep into some part of her being. Into her soul if I could stretch it just a bit more. Because that's how it seemed.

Then she started crying. Just like that. Crying really hard.
And she never took her eyes off the mirror.
She never took her eyes off her soul.

I am a trained registered nurse. I have seen trauma and death. I have seen humanity at it's worst…and it's best. I am a compassionate fellow and pretty good at helping people in their neediest moments. But I was totally frozen. I had no freakin' idea what I should do…or if I should do anything.

She cried for about 30 seconds. Nonstop. Tears. Sobs. Her gaze never left the mirror. Her gaze never left her soul and I swear to goodness that with each sob she seemed to grow a little more determined. Almost as if she was preparing for something.

I didn't know what.

Then she stopped. Just like that.

She washed her face…patted it dry with a towel. Put on just a bit of make-up. Not a lot. Folded the towel, grabbed her small bag and walked out. The door slowly started to close behind her.

Like a strange dream, as soon as the door closed behind her it immediately re-opened and my morning crew of five RN's and charge nurse walked in. It was as if the previous 12 minutes existed only in my mind.

Little did I know how much my life had just changed. Forever.

The night crew signed off, the day crew, us, signed in and hit the floor to go meet our patients. I gotta say I was excited. Excited because of where I was and who I was caring for. I had my patient list in my hand…room 302…turned the corner…there's the room…knock-knock…come in…I opened the door and began to introduce myself as Lieutenant Martinez…and I froze.

The lady from the lounge. She was my first patient's mother. He…Well…He was a young man who lost a limb…an eye… part of one ear…and his mom was at his side. The same five foot nothing lady from the lounge who I had just seen.

She greeted me with a smile and a thank you for taking care of her son and it was then that I realized the absolute power of the mind and all it can give us…all it can offer us…and all we can take from it IF we just learn to harness it in the right way.

This mom, who started off my 18-month tour at Walter Reed Army Medical Center, woke up every single day with the same routine. She cried in the same place. She let it all out before walking into her son's room each and every morning because she knew she had to be strong for two people – for her, …and for her son.

There was an easy road…I'm sure. To ask God why…to cry in front of her boy…to let the environment take control…to just quit…to give up. But she chose to take control of her environment. She chose to control her situation. She made the conscious decision each and every day for the many months they were there…to take charge of her day… of her life. She woke up and set her mind.

I got to know her and her son. They both healed. They both

overcame their obstacles and they both became better people… changed for their experience.

THE SOLUTION

How does this help you? Other than the story about the experience…how does this help you achieve a better body? Learn to eat better. How does it help you…the reader, learn to set your mind on your goals. To develop the *mindset* we all need to get over life's daily hurdles. I can describe it in one simple sentence, and then I'll break it into a series of 5 simple steps to achieve the *mindset* to WIN everyday.

The one simple sentence?

Because you owe it to yourself to be the best possible version of yourself and that battle starts each and every day.

She wasn't an athlete. She wasn't an icon. She was a mom.

Think about that for a second.

I came to see and then describe the things that made that mom win each and every day. I would say that she developed habits. Because habits then became part of who she was. And as I prepared to leave Walter Reed and enter the world of physical fitness, coaching and motivating people, I developed a simple series of steps that I then began to follow. Then to teach. …And now to share with you.

They are rather simple…because simplicity is genius in my opinion and they flow as such:

    Step 1: Define your goals

    Step 2: Evaluate yourself

    Step 3: Decide on your program/regimen

    Step 4: Start your program/regimen

    Step 5: Reassess yourself after 4 weeks

Step 1. **Write** it down.
Make sure it is important to you. Put it on your bathroom mirror. "I want to be a better mom"…"I want to lose 8 pounds"…"I never again want to be the fat dad on the sidelines of my kids games." Write it down and make it visible. Then look at it each and every day. Burn it into your soul each morning.

Step 2. **Evaluate** yourself.
Yeah, I said that. Take a picture of yourself with an iPhone. Get on a scale and get your weight. Don't be embarrassed, just do it. Your neighbor didn't force feed you Twinkies so don't blame anyone but yourself if the numbers on the scale are not to your liking. Write down for one full week everything you put into your piehole. Evaluate yourself folks. And be honest. And last thing? Get a journal and prepare to track how you look, how you feel and how you perform each day.

Step 3. **Decide** on your program.
The message here? Do something. Order P-90X. Go to a Cross-Fit gym. Join Anytime Fitness. Go for a walk everyday. Just please start moving you body. The other 80% of the program? Nutrition. Eat clean and eat for life…Por Vida! In a sentence, eat meat, veggies, nuts and seeds, some fruit, little starch and NO sugar. Decide on your program and stick to it.

Step 4. **Start.**
Go. Begin. Move. Take immediate action for 30 solid days to develop new habits and begin to alter your lifestyle. Folks this is important. We must follow the regimen we set out to do for at least 30 days so it becomes a part of who we are. So it becomes a part of our being. It starts with day one. And guess what. It's not easy. Think about what the mom faced…then think about what you face. Any excuses? Didn't think so.

Step 5. **Reassess.**
Your 30-day assessment. Don't do a 30-day assessment if you haven't stuck to days 1-29. Seriously. Don't kid yourself. If you've soul searched and you have stuck to a plan or regimen or

program for days 1-29, then do this. Look at your journal.

What are your wins? Perhaps you are doing more pushups. Maybe eating better five times a week as opposed to zero times per week.

What are your hurdles? Review you journal and see where you were stuck. Maybe it was Friday nights because all the gals got together for "Chardonnay Night."

How can you continue to get better? Review your wins and review your hurdles and start to dig into how you can be even better.

There you have it. A story about frame of mind. A five-step plan. A breakout of each of the five steps for 30 days.

EPILOGUE

Before I left Washington, D.C. there was a parade. It went right down Constitution Avenue. I rode my bike and walked through the crowd. It was Veterans Day. The parade procession went by...heroes...guys with US flags on Harleys...bands...and then it was him. My patient. The same one from day one. I could tell, by his face that his mind...was set.

No excuses. Our hurdles will rarely ever be as tough as theirs.

Go.
Win.
Now.

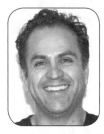

About Rick

Rick Martinez is a registered nurse by degree and an entrepreneur at heart. Having started his first company in 2001, MedTrust, LLC, he went on to form Fitness Porvida, LLC in 2007 after a life changing experience working with amputees at Walter Reed Army Medical Center as an Army nurse in 2006.

In 2011 Rick sold his company to focus on his passion of becoming a catalyst for change in health and fitness in his local and greater communities, and also giving back to the Americans who protect our freedoms.

Fitness Porvida, or "For Life" is the battle cry of the growing Tribe of faithful followers in his home of San Antonio, Texas.

Awards and accomplishments include:

- San Antonio's "40 Under 40"
- Awarded the prestigious Jefferson Award for community service
- Recognized as one of the country's "Top 100 Companies" by the US Small Business Administration
- Awarded "Best of the City" for health clubs. First ever CrossFit gym to receive this award
- Raised $71,000 for Special Operation Warrior Foundation in a one day event

Rick has been featured on ABC, NBC, CBS and Fox affiliates as San Antonio's 'fitness expert' and has published several articles in local and national journals related to health, wellness and on how to look better naked.

Rick is married to Lisa, his wife of over 10 years and has three wonderful, healthy kids. Katelyn, Kelsey and Slaton. Actually, five kids if you count his two Labs, Mookie and Murphy.

"With much humility, I believe my passion in this life is to help people realize their dreams. Whether they be in fitness, in life or in business, I feel I have been given this one opportunity on earth to make as much of a difference as I can for anyone who will choose to listen, and I refuse to squander it. My experience is no different…no grander and no more special than anyone else's. I was shaped by my simple upbringings and my parents, by my service in the Army, by my family, by my wins and losses, by my involvement with Entrepreneurs Organization (EO), and by God. Everyday I'm hustling."

The guy to call when you wanna look better naked.

To learn more about Rick, his organization or his mission, check out:
www.fitnessporvida.com
rick@fitnessporvida.com

CHAPTER 5

Seven Simple Steps to Guarantee Success

By Jolene Goring

What would you say if I told you that I would share seven simple steps that would guarantee success in any part of your life? Would you be interested to know what they were? Of course you would! If you wish to improve any area of your life, then read on... and be prepared for your life to change in any way that you desire – the sky is the limit!

There is one thing in common that all successful people do. What is it? They all employ the same basic principles to achieve their goals. Almost every person who has achieved success in any area of their life has followed the same seven principles that I am going to share with you. Doesn't it make sense to follow the lead of others who are flourishing, and leverage their trial- and-error to your advantage? There is no need to reinvent the wheel, when the formula for success is laid out right in front of you.

The concepts that you will learn to implement are: goal setting, making a timeline and action plan, accountability, evaluation, flexibility and rewarding yourself. These sound like simple ideas and they are. When these simple seven steps are put together in the proper sequence, they become extremely effective at paving the path for you to achieve your goals!

These seven steps can be applied to any area of your life, but for the context of this book we will stay in the fitness realm. Realistically, without good health you will not be able to achieve and maintain success in other areas of your life. It makes perfect sense to set your first and most important goal to obtain better health. Now, better health could mean many things to different people, but the commonality of good health is unlimited! More energy, a positive outlook on life, more productivity, less stress, better sleep, greater happiness, more sex appeal, higher libido, prevention of new health problems and combatting existing health conditions - these and many, many more benefits can be achieved simply by committing to achieving better health. And how does one do this? By following the seven simple steps outlined below. These steps are not difficult, but they do require dedication. You have to WANT and BELIEVE in your goal. If you have the desire, here is the strategy. Are you ready? Let's go!

1. Set specific goals.

It is not enough to have a goal to 'lose weight.' What does that mean – one pound or 100 pounds? The more specific that you are, the greater your chances of success are. If you want to build muscle, you can keep track of the amount of weights that you use, and monitor the increase in weight and / or reps that you can do. If you want to fit into your 'skinny jeans' then hang them where you can see them every day. Whatever your goal is, cut out magazine photos of your ideal body, and create a vision board. By having a daily reminder of what you are working towards, you will be more motivated to stay on track and keep moving in the right direction. The more effort you put into defining your goal, the more realistic it will feel, and the more attainable it will be. As Walt Disney says: "If you can dream it, you can do it!"

2. Make a timeline.

Once you decide on your ultimate goal – break it down into smaller steps. The thought of losing 50 pounds can be daunting, but if you make a smaller goal to lose 2 pounds this week, that is very attainable. The most successful people create timelines for achieving their goals. These timelines contain both weekly and monthly objectives. Start at your ultimate goal and work backwards to break the large goal into smaller pieces. This will help you to see the small steps that you will need to take, in order to achieve your larger goal.

3. Create an action plan.

This is a common stumbling block for many people – once you know WHAT you want to achieve, you need to plan exactly HOW you are going to achieve your goal. How many people do you know who talk about doing something, but then never actually follow through? The majority of people are all talk and no action. This is not because people don't want to achieve their goals. The reason is that most people don't have a clear plan of action towards their goal. They may think that they are working in the right direction, but if they haven't planned their action out properly then they could be doing a lot of work for nothing. Don't be one of those people – set a specific plan of action and do it! Identify what specific steps are necessary for you to achieve both your smaller and larger goals. Also make note of anything that may get in the way of your achieving your objectives, and plan on how you will overcome these obstacles. By planning all of this out in advance, it will be infinitely easier for you to keep moving in the direction of your dreams no matter what life throws at you!

4. Be accountable.

This is the single most important step for success. Tell your colleagues that you are making healthy changes. Get your friends and family onside. Hire a personal trainer to keep you on track. The more people that know about your goals, the higher your chance of success to achieve them! For example, if you tell your colleague that your goal is to lose 2 pounds this week, you will likely think twice before you eat a doughnut during that morning meeting. You now feel accountable to her because you know that she is watching you. You can even ask close friends to help you monitor your daily habits – many people mindlessly snack and may not even be aware of it! You could offer to give friends and family a dollar for every time they catch you doing something that is not in line with your goal. <u>The bottom line is that the more people that are motivating and helping you to achieve your goal, the greater your chance of success!</u>

5. Evaluate.

This step is different for everyone. For some people, spending 2 minutes every evening reflecting on their day is the best way for them to evaluate their progress. Other people prefer to check in with themselves on a weekly basis. The key is to not wait longer than a week to evaluate your progress. This will make sure that you stay on track. If you have deviated from your plan of action, you can easily get back on track without too much effort. For example, if your goal is to compete in a marathon, do a weekly assessment of your distance, time, and how you feel. Based on this analysis, you can make any necessary changes to your action plan. This will allow you to tweak your program immediately if something is not working. Don't expect everything to work out perfectly the first time you make your action plan and then evaluate a week later – it will likely take a few weeks to make adjustments to where you are making the most improvements. As you get bigger / better/ faster / stronger... you will need to keep making adjustments to your action plan to continue advancing towards your ultimate goal.

6. Have flexibility.

The most important element to making lasting lifestyle

changes is to learn to live a healthy life for the long term, not to make unrealistic short-term lifestyle changes. For example, if you are going on a beach vacation, you will not be able to do your regular gym workout with your trainer. This is not a reason to take the week off from fitness - you need to improvise a new and fun way to stay active on the trip! You can run on the beach, use rocks as weights instead of dumbells, do pushups and lunges on the sand, swim in the water... the possibilities are endless! By being flexible yet disciplined with your routine, you will be able to keep your healthy habits no matter what life throws at you.

Being flexible will help with your success when work gets in the way of your health goal. If you get stuck with a big work project and are having a hard time fitting your regular fitness routine in, you will have to be creative. In this case you will need to block out a chunk of time for yourself, and treat it like an important business meeting. Maybe you prefer to work out first thing in the morning, but because of a big project you have to be at work too early to work out. It would be easy to say that you have no time to work out, but you are better than that! <u>You always have choices</u> - you can either go to bed earlier so that you can get up earlier, or you can decide that your lunch hour will be your new gym time. The bottom line is that with a little flexibility, creativity, and smart choices, there is no excuse to not pursue your healthy goals!

7. Reward yourself.

When you lose your first 2 pounds – treat yourself! Set aside a half hour to do an indulgent 'waste of time' activity that you enjoy but that you never make the time to do. John Lennon states it best: "Time you enjoy wasting, was not wasted." Maybe you choose to indulge in reading a trashy celebrity magazine, or watching your favorite TV show, or even just sitting and doing absolutely nothing.

The key is to enjoy your time; you have earned it! By rewarding yourself in a healthy and enjoyable way, you are setting positive reinforcement that healthy habits result in good things. For your larger monthly milestone achievements, plan greater rewards such as going to a movie with a friend, buying that pair of shoes you have been eyeing, or something else that you find special.

If you follow these seven simple tips, you will be guaranteed to reach any and all of your health and fitness goals!

Once you have your health in check, you are ready to apply the above seven steps to other areas of your life. It is useful to choose one area of your life at a time to focus on, so that you do not get overwhelmed. Now that you have great health, you can achieve anything that you desire! The most difficult part will be deciding what area of your life you want to improve next: relationships, career, spirituality, or studies - absolutely any part of your life can be improved by following the seven steps above. *The key is to never stop growing, and never stop reaching for the stars!*

Hopefully you will <u>pay your success forward</u> by inspiring someone else to take their health into their own hands. There is no better feeling than to help someone achieve a higher level of health, and you now have the tools to encourage another person to feel as great as you do … Congratulations!

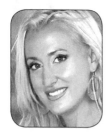

About Jolene

Jolene Goring is a leading health and fitness expert based in Scottsdale, AZ. She has been featured in USA Today, and is a regular contributor to the Fitness Expert Network. She is also a featured personal trainer in various fitness videos.

Jolene has been involved in the health and fitness industry for 12 years. She has taught yoga on the beach in Mexico, studied belly dancing in Egypt, traveled the world as a fitness model, taught snowboarding in Canada, and studied yoga in an ashram in India. She has trained with personal trainers and participated in extreme sports worldwide. She has her Bachelor of Science degree, and numerous health, nutrition, and fitness certifications. Jolene is always looking for new challenges, and her next big adventures will be hiking to the base camp of Everest, and learning how to skydive!

Jolene is the Fitness Director of Geo-Fit, an exclusive personal training company based in Scottsdale, AZ. Geo-Fit utilizes different fitness techniques from around the world, to provide the most fun, effective, and safest workouts available.

Jolene trains clients one-on-one, in group settings, and via phone worldwide. Call 480-510-5305 for a FREE in person or telephone consult, or email: info@geo-fit.com. Visit: www.geo-fit.com for your FREE *"Exclusive Scottsdale Fat Loss Plan"*.

www.geo-fit.com

CHAPTER 6

Bigger, Better, Stronger, and Faster with the Right Mindset

By Stacy Ward

I remember as a small child having big dreams. I always felt like I would make a big difference one day in the world. My parents divorced when I was 6 years-old and I endured a lot of mental personal struggles through my youth and teenage years. My big dreams and self-worth started to slowly fade away. I had major fears of abandonment and started to allow other people's views and opinions of me mold me and matter more than my own. Looking back, all my beliefs about love, happiness, health, success were shattered and I allowed the negativity around me to take hold of me and I would play those recordings in my head over and over.

I thankfully went to a military high school where discipline and physical education were very important. I was more motivated when others were counting on me and I loved the camaraderie of team sports. Working together with others sharing a common goal and feeling a part of something helped me out of the negativity that I felt as a teen. Sports gave me my self-confidence and taught me self-discipline through practicing each day, and perseverance to never give up during game time – no matter how far we were behind. I learned that even when our team wasn't as skilled as the other teams that we could still win if we truly believed and if our desire to win was greater than the opponents.

I learned success is deliberate through having a vision, creating a plan of action, rehearsing and practicing that plan, having a good coach to push you harder and keeping you focused were important. I learned perseverance and patience. I learned that sometimes I will fail, but to learn from my failures and my mistakes – in order to improve and make me better.

A huge turning point for me in my life was learning that I am not a failure when I fail, unless I allowed that failure to stop me from pursuing my goal.

So how does this story relate to you and help you! After years of experiences in my life and working with clients as a fitness trainer and coach, I have discovered the 4 Steps to help you create a mindset for change that can help you Think Bigger, Become Better, Grow Stronger, and Act Faster!

FOUR STEPS TO CREATE CHANGE
IN MINDSET FOR SUCCESS

First, start thinking of yourself as an athlete, that life is a game and how you can play to win the game. You might be thinking well, I'm not an athlete, so let's address this first principle. Belief...

I learned this the hard way. If you don't believe in yourself or your ability to reach your goal, you will never see success. Small time thinking will never lead to Bigger Dreams. Your core beliefs about who you are will determine your actions no matter how great the plan is. So you must address this first. For example, you can take two people, give them the exact same perfect plan for success, and only one will succeed. Why? Is it because one person is better than the other, has better genetics or their life is predetermined for success, or they are lucky! Mostly likely not! The difference is the one who believes will succeed because they have mastered a secret that I will share.

Let's dig in to our core beliefs! Our core beliefs are usually shaped around childhood and can change over time. Our experiences and how we perceive them will mold our core beliefs. How people react to us and how we react to situations start to create a pattern of belief that is either healthy or unhealthy. If we place our life experiences on a balance scale with one side good experiences and the other side bad experiences, and over time the tipping scale is filled with bad experiences or unhealthy perceptions, our life will become unbalanced. Our mental outlook will project the side of the heaviest. The heaviest side of the scale is where our experiences in this life have spent the most time and those experiences have been reinforced over and over again. Like a mental recording that gets played over and over again. Those mental recordings are played subconsciously whenever we make decisions. They are the head coaches in our game of life. Sometimes *we have to fire that head coach* if we are going to win the game in life!

STEP ONE — THINK BIGGER VISION

Have a Bigger Dream!

If you are dreaming small, chances are, you don't think of yourself as someone who is worthy or capable. Visualize the big dream even if you don't think it is possible. The old saying fake it until you make it applies; therefore, see yourself as you having already succeeded in your mind. Next, work on your weaknesses by identifying them and enlist the help of a coach or someone who has strengths in your areas of weakness. Practice skills and habits that will cultivate better outcomes. Break down these skills into something manageable or smaller, and master them. Once you start improving and mastering them yourself, confidence will improve and will take some of the weight off the scale.

STEP TWO — BECOME BETTER AT
HAVING A BETTER GAME

Having a Better Game requires practice. We all know practice makes perfect, however, have realistic expectations and understand that there will be setbacks and obstacles along the way. After identifying core beliefs and weaknesses, we have to look at our failures or weaknesses and improve them or practice them in order to get better. For example, if we only practice the skills that we are good at, will we become better? If we only train the body part that we like to train, will we improve the part that is weak? No, the same is true for our mindset. The one thing I tell my clients is that the ones who persevere during setbacks are the ones who will successfully achieve their goals. If you look at the most successful people in life, the ones who are achieving what you want to achieve – they weren't always winners.

For example, Oprah Winfrey endured an abusive childhood and numerous setbacks including getting fired from a job as a TV reporter because she was unfit for TV. Along with being the most prolific homerun hitter, Babe Ruth had more strikeouts than anyone else - His quote: "Every strike brings me closer to the next home run." Walt Disney was fired by a newspaper editor because he said he lacked imagination and didn't have good ideas. The one thing all these people have in common is that they have all failed, they never gave up their dream, and they used their failure to learn how to be better. Every failure was a gift to grow Stronger. I believe we all have a gift to share to the world and it may not be as big as these examples, but it is equally important. If you give up, not only will you never see success, you will also take away the precious gifts you were given to show the world.

STEP THREE — GROW STRONGER
— GET OUT OF COMFORT ZONES AND
DEVELOP MENTAL TOUGHNESS

We grow stronger by getting out of our comfort zones and getting rid of the fear that holds us hostage to unrealized dreams.

It is impossible for someone who has fear of failure to achieve anything, because they never try. They never give themselves the opportunity to succeed because they have already said in their mind that they can't. My clients all know how I hate the word 'can't' which may slip out of their mouths when they are pushing themselves out of their comfort zones. Every circumstance that it slips out of their mouth during a workout, they always prove that they can if they put their mind to it. Don't confuse 'can't' with 'won't' because you always can but you may not want to. It is in doing, trying and experiencing things you have never done before, getting out of those comfort zones, where you will grow stronger – and with practice you will get better and better at things you do. Just like a muscle that you want stronger. You apply a bigger force in order to break it down and rebuild it to make it stronger. This truth is applied to everything in life.

So in our game of life, we must undergo big life experiences that may seem at the time to really break us down mentally, physically, and spiritually. Those life experiences are, in my opinion, treasures. In those experiences we learn the most about ourselves, seek deeper meaning of life. We can all transform those experiences and create a better life and a better game.

Mental toughness is something all good coaches strive to teach their players. Having all the talent in the world means nothing when it comes to game time if you haven't practiced and mastered your thoughts. If self-doubt is going through your mind, your game will suffer. If you were standing at the batter's box and life is throwing you a curve ball, and self-doubt took over your mind and you were worried about striking out, do you think you could hit a home run? Cultivating a stronger and better belief in yourself and your ability is the only way you will succeed and hit the homerun in life!

Here is an affirmation that I use to help me when I have self-doubt or fear of failing that may help you if you are struggling with this.

"Every failure brings me closer to experiencing a better life."

How to step out of your comfort zone:

Start by doing the things that you are fearful of. Looking fear in the eye and say "bring it on!" If you realize that failing can be a recipe for success as long as you persevere, then you will not fear failing. If you demolish in your mind the fear of failing you will not be afraid of trying. It is in the process of trying something new that you start to experience a new life. If you want to change self-sabotaging behavior, you have got to have the courage to change and learn to blow through obstacles in your path. Whenever we are faced with an obstacle or setback, our defense mechanism will revert back to the way that is most comfortable. Our bodies view stressful situations with a fight-or-flight mechanism. If you have a lifetime of experiences with running away from the problems or reverting back to your old patterns because that is what is familiar and comfortable, the new change is different and the body views it as stressful. It will send warning signals; this could be dangerous, so flee. However, you have to fight through those setbacks in order to win the battle and create a positive lasting lifestyle change and win the game of life. This is why only the top 5-10% of people are successful in their weight loss journey, career life, and athletic performance.

Most people want change; they want to look good, feel good, perform better, and have a purpose-filled life with meaning. However, the majority of the population do not want to get out of their comfort zone and experience new thoughts and a different way of living. We are creatures of habit. Our daily habits determine our designation in life. How fast we respond to difficulties in life and make changes will ultimately lead us to a shorter or longer path to success.

STEP FOUR — ACT FASTER – HIRE A GOOD COACH – BREAK DOWN GOALS IN FAST ACTION STEPS

Looking at an athlete's speed, how fast they can get from point A to point B and how fast they can think and react to circumstance, will determine if they beat their opponent.

If you need help, hire a coach and break down your goals into fast action steps. Your coach will help you set goals that are S.M.A.R.T. – Specific, Measurable, Attainable, Realistic, and Timely.

We develop confidence in ourselves when we accomplish goals. We start gaining confidence to try new things when we start accomplishing and creating good experiences, and that scale of life starts to tip the other way with more good experiences and perceptions. Momentum is built by speed of actions. You must act quickly or self-doubt will enter in. People become frozen without action because they over analyze situations. Once you know what you want and have the right plan to act, don't fall victim to procrastination. There is never the right time to start. If you find yourself making more excuses why you can't now, then guess what? You will never see success. Procrastination is just another way to say "I am fearful of failure, so I don't want to start."

Once you learn these techniques of seeing an obstacle or a setback as a positive thing, you will move faster toward your goal with bullet speed. If you establish short goals that you can accomplish quickly, you will find that you will move along that long path towards your vision mentally much faster, with more motivation and confidence. Once you master your first goal, move to another one that moves you forward. You can always find a way to move forward even during periods where outside forces may get in the way. Create a path around them and problem solve. If you aren't a good problem solver, a good coach can help you create a path around. Even if you feel you are only making small insignificant changes…those changes are changing daily habits. Those daily habits are important in the big scheme of things.

BEING IN THE ZONE —
BRINGING IT ALL TOGETHER

Being in the zone is a term that athletes use when everything they have practiced is being played out perfectly in a game situation. It is working in the flow where your senses are heightened, everything is in slow motion, every obstacle in your path is blown away perfectly. You feel energized and inspired, and it feels like a perfect dream. It is effortless! It is a moment that after you have it, that you strive for. You are thankful, live with gratitude, have a positive outlook and want to share it with others.

Why is this important to strive for?

It is important because, through your transformation, you can help transform society and those around you. As a society, when every person can transform their mindset to Think Bigger, Feel Better, Grow Stronger, and Act Faster, we can collectively improve our game in this life and help others by showing them that it is possible – because I did it and so can you!

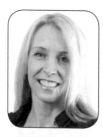

About Stacy

Stacy has been in the health and fitness industry for 15 years. Passionately helping thousands of people get in shape, eat better, and change their lifestyle. She has a degree in Exercise Science, and is certified as a personal trainer, boot camp instructor, nutrition coach, and wellness coach. She has also recently appeared in the TV show "Meet The Experts" and featured in USA Today as America's Premier Fitness Expert.

She incorporates her integrated style approach to helping clients create a lifestyle change that addresses her five principle foundations for lasting transformation. After working in health clubs for over 10 years and watching the high turnover of employees and drop out rates of new members, she wanted to reach out to those whose needs were not being met in that atmosphere.

Her company STA-FIT Health Solutions & Fit Body Boot Camp was created to address the needs of those who are frustrated with their lack of results. She has created lifestyle programs that offer a way to challenge the mind, body, and spirit through educating her clients with proper goal setting, addressing sabotaging behaviors, creating a plan and a solution with proper nutrition, supplementation, and exercise – all while holding them accountable through group and individual accountability programs.

She offers customized solutions for those who need more attention with one-to-one personal services in home or in private studio, as well as group training to address a larger audience who prefer to engage in a dynamic group environment. Her strong desire to help as many people as possible was the driving force behind her boot camp business.

Her mission is to use her business to be the vehicle that moves her clients forward on their journey towards better health and a better life with a balanced approach. Her vision is to create a different lifestyle approach for people that will help them be more productive at work, have more energy, happy with the way they look, help them connect with others who share common goal, and empower her clients to share their stories – to make a difference in the community and in their homes as good role models. Her motto is "lead by example!" As a busy mother, dedicated wife and business owner, she strives to continue her journey of spiritual growth, living with the purpose of making a difference, balancing her own healthy living, while also empowering clients with a deeper purpose in mind.

Stacy is taking steps to reach out into the community and give to those in need by working with local food bank, church, and charity events. She motivates her clients to use their increased fitness to also give back through being fit to serve others, participating in races for local charity, other fitness events, and mission trips. Her company hosts annual community events like "Burn the Fat to Feed the Hungry" – which is a food drive for a local food bank, and last year her boot campers raised over $5,000 to help Wounded Warriors in Woodstock, GA. with the local fire and police department.

Her company services Canton, Woodstock, and Roswell, Georgia and can be reached at: www.stayfitwithstacy.com or www.fitbodybootcampga.com for free trial.

CHAPTER 7

The Recipe for Success and Getting Started

By Joe Green, CPFT, CNC, CES

How important is to you to change the way you feel and make it last for a lifetime? Many have trouble accepting success, much like accepting a compliment. Are you able to receive a compliment and graciously accept it with thanks? Can you see yourself successfully reaching your goals... whether it's dropping two waist sizes, running that 5K marathon or even just getting back that sexy attractive feeling of self-worth and appeal?

If you've struggled or had to start over more than once and you've fallen short of your goals, then the information in this book is a gold mine. But nothing, and I mean nothing will work if you're not ready to do what it takes, and to do it the right way. I want you to imagine what it would feel like to set out to reach your goals, knowing that this time is the last time you're ever going to have to start over. That's right, I'm talking about succeeding once and for all, and at the end of the journey working on maintaining your results or maybe setting new goals.

It all begins here at the start, day one. I think it's fair to say that everyone starts with the best of intentions. Are you ready to learn more about fitness and your personality, in other words who you are today? Are you looking to not only get healthy and fit, but to also embrace your new found health and fitness as a new lifestyle and make it last forever?

Becoming healthy and fit is a process of great transformation and change. The successful journey involves a change in the way you think and feel. It involves getting in touch with your motivations and your challenges in a way that you may not be familiar with. Grasp this approach and the concepts to follow and you will solve the mystery, you'll remove the thin veil of disguise and find the answers and the ultimate solution to success that everyone's seeking.

What's the secret to getting healthy and fit and making it last?

We have three aspects to our general well being, and all three must be "in working order" if you truly want to grasp a hold of success, and maintain it for any real sustained period of time.

You have to get your Healthy House in order, in other words you have to get healthy from the inside out. Both exercise and nutrition are emotional experiences. Fact is, life is an emotional experience, and our collection of past experiences has a lot to do with how we go about succeeding and how we feel about ourselves today.

This is very powerful information. If I can get you to understand this concept, embrace it, solve it and use it to your absolute pure benefit... You win... and the fit, healthy, happy lifestyle you've been searching for will be yours. Skip this exercise (no pun intended) and you will spin your wheels in place endlessly. My goal is to help you break that cycle of self-sabotage and destruction – once and for all.

We talk about creating a new lifestyle yet most are defeated before they even start, just because:

1. The methods they have chosen are actually harmful and even injurious.

2. The road to any success they've had has been scattered and a hodgepodge of advice and ideas.

THE RECIPE FOR SUCCESS AND GETTING STARTED

3. They chose short-term quick results (not a life-style) change for now <u>and</u> for the future.

Why are these approaches so unsuccessful? Let's take a moment and break down the flaws so that if one of the three pitfalls above presents itself, you won't end up on the casualty list.

First! Most popular methods of self-sabotage leading to fleeting temporary results is that the method or means used towards accomplishing health and fitness goals cause injury – resulting in repeated frustrating setbacks.

For example, setting a goal of running five miles today and one mile more per day for the next few weeks or so when you haven't run that distance in years is a poor choice of goals, and the approach is likely suited for injury and/or failure. And we all know how frustrating setbacks can be.

Remember, the way you achieve your results plays a large part in what it will take to maintain those same results. Taking an approach like this is a real bust!

Second! One of the most notorious goal assassins of all time... Not having a system, which leads to lack-of-focus, and ultimately failure. The majority of us are so desperate, frustrated and confused with a ton of questions... How do I lose weight? ... What should I eat for breakfast or after a workout? ...How much protein should I eat? ...How often should I exercise? <gulp of air> ...Is there a limit to how much cardio I should do to burn fat vs. muscle? Can I lose fat and gain muscle at any age? Can women really get bulky from weight training? ...Are the supplements I take potentially fatal? Phew! ... And the list goes on and on of questions and concerns. Suspect food labels, supplements, exercise gadgets and more, all deliver empty promises – which add to all of the confusion. No doubt everyone has an opinion, but there is only one truth.

So many turn to friends, those who "look" like they know better or even to magazines, ads and infomercials that make unrealistic claims. Heck, the gym seems like a logical place to go, but most often it's merely a dead end dangling the promise of a carrot you'll never reach, let alone taste.

Often this approach results in a blend of hearsay-advice from others, what you've read in magazines along with a heaping dose of enticing infomercial ads mixed with fad-diet promises. This hodgepodge approach usually brings about results that are scattered and almost always fleeting, the true recipe for continued doom and frustration!

Third! One of the most repeated guaranteed failing methods going. The only winners in this one are the marketers who prey upon you. Enticing ads promising quick, fast results actually lure in the general public by the thousands – on a daily and repeated basis.

Fad diets and gadgets advertised on television continually sell out, failing to deliver "lasting" results. These empty promises lead you to another dead end. The real crime of it all is that many consumers believe that they failed to succeed at making proper use of the advertised solution or product when in fact the solution or product itself is ineffective to begin with. Read that last sentence back, it's the truth and it's just one of the "ah-ha" moments to be found amongst the pages of this book.

There are no quick fixes nor should we be looking for any. A real lifestyle change is about the long run, not just for the here and now. It's a new way of living the rest of your life. So what's it take, what is the key to real, long lasting results that do more than just address what we see in the mirror? How do we get healthy from the inside out, so that we feel as healthy and vibrant as ever?

It takes the right approach. You must get your "Healthy House" in order. Combined with a program customized to meet your needs, challenges and goals, all you need to do is to incorporate what I call the Three House Rules and that is the ultimate key –

the recipe for success. Sounds simple, yet we just talked about three of the most popular downfalls that sabotage so many:

- Ineffective methodologies that cause injury and repeated setbacks.
- Chaos and mass confusion which produces scattered results and completely waists your time and money, and
- Quick fixes linked to empty promises that never really pan out.

USE THESE 3 RULES AND PROSPER

Here are three rules that lead to the kind of richly rewarding and long lasting success in health and fitness that everyone is searching for:

1. Personal Blueprint
2. Psychological Connection
3. Physical Focus

Let's go through a brief exercise to help you create and organize a healthy and fit lifestyle program that really helps you get started and on the right track. I'm going to empower you and give you the control that you absolutely have to have to succeed.

HOUSE RULE #1 – PERSONAL BLUEPRINT

The first house rule addresses the personal aspect of you achieving the health and fitness you have been searching for. You have to build a strong foundation and it starts right here with this all-important step of addressing your personal being.

Grab a notebook, this is a healthy exercise for helping you to journal or in other words, document your path to success. Later it will be the road map that you look back on, serving as your moral compass to keep you on track or when needed to get you back on track. Remember that a dream is just a dream until it is committed to paper.

So here we go, answer the questions slowly and honestly. If you find yourself stuck then the process is working, and if you find yourself spilling out answers without much trouble, then the process is working. You can't lose with this exercise.

1. What are your health and fitness goals and how important is it to you to reach these goals?

2. What is your vision, what would it look like and feel like to succeed at reaching your personal goals?

3. Do you give yourself the permission to succeed?

4. Do you have a personal mission statement? (If not, create one now.)

I can't want your goals more than you do, in fact no one else can. You have to want it most of all and it has to be for your own personal reasons. You shouldn't have to be sick to take your health, your time, your energy and all of your other valuable resources seriously. You're worth it.

HOUSE RULE #2 – PSYCHOLOGICAL CONNECTION

The second house rule deals with the psychological aspect of achieving your health and fitness goals once and for all. Make no mistake, this is the golden key among the three because herein rests the real power to make the necessary changes and strides towards success.

No one makes it and in fact many fail because this piece is not whole and healthy. The mind is more than just a terrible thing to waste. It's a terrible thing to underestimate. Your mind and the emotions and feelings you have about yourself, your life, your family, your career and your dreams are all hard wired to your ability to succeed and reach your goals. You are what you think you are, and you can be the best version of what you want to be if you allow yourself. We encourage our children to reach for the stars and to dream, and we motivate them to believe. So let's get back to basics, you have to start believing in yourself.

Believe me when I tell you how absolutely necessary this exercise is. You must get in touch with your mind and make the connection to what it is you really want. Failure to do this is the reason why celebrities on down to the person next door fail to succeed. Let's get started with the five questions below and remember to take your time with this. Time is the first essential investment that you will make in yourself and one of the most valuable.

1. What makes you happy? (Explain)

2. What motivates you? (Explain)

3. Describe yourself in 10 words?

4. What are the things you would like to change most about yourself? (Explain)

5. Describe what a "healthy and fit you" looks and feels like? (Explain)

Honor and explore the capabilities and abilities you have and where they are coming from. In order to have vision, you need light to travel by. Turn on the lights by stimulating your thought process with this exercise. Remember that if your mind isn't in it, then believe me my friend, your heart isn't either. This is another important building block in the process of creating a new bigger, better, faster, stronger you.

HOUSE RULE #3 – PHYSICAL FOCUS

The third house rule organizes the physical aspect of your health and fitness success by putting you in a position to succeed. Sounds simple but many set themselves up for failure with this step alone. Don't become another New Year's resolution statistic. Your fitness program should be custom designed with built in factors sure to fuel your motivation and success. Go through and answer the questions below to get yourself pointed in the right direction.

1. What time of day will you exercise and where will you go? (Have to like it.)

2. What gets you pumped and ready to roll? (Music, atmosphere, workout partner…)

3. What is your fitness personality? (Prefer weights, one-on-one, classes, running…)

4. Consider your past medical history and present condition? (Injuries, chronic pain, surgeries, medicines, etc.)

Customize your approach and make certain that your goals are realistic and as healthy as the results you desire. Make sure you consult with your doctor to help make healthy choices that are just right for you.

Congratulations, you've just created your own personal blueprint to be the best you can possibly be. Read it back and get your Healthy House organized and in order – so that you have a rock solid foundation to build on. You can do it, I believe in you!

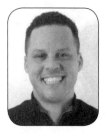

About Joe

Joe Green, CPFT, CNC, CES is the Founder and Owner of Fit For You. Joe's philosophies, training methodology and tools are at the leading edge of performance training with a focus on a simple foundation and premise for exercise variety intended to affect steady and consistent progress over time.

Joe is a trusted and highly-regarded resource of the medical community including some world-renowned facilities for his work with special populations facing movement disorders, chronic illness and post-therapy rehabilitation. His medically-supervised programs are at the forefront of the revolution on making fitness a successful and healthy lifestyle that can and will truly last a lifetime thereby dismissing the inefficient, dangerous and injurious training methodologies of the past. With his evolving programs, educational seminars and a growing network of medical professionals, the opportunity to see and feel the future of health and fitness exists at Fit For You. In fact, the collaborative and mutually supportive bond that exists between Joe Green and the medical community has yielded some of the best long-term results available today.

Fit For You also offers highly specialized programs designed to benefit women, youthful athletes and recreational sports participants.

For more information on the highly skilled services and programs offered, please go to: www.phyt4u.com

CHAPTER 8

Seeing is Believing -
The Mental Side of Fitness Success

By Mike Bevard

When people come to me wanting to lose weight, oftentimes all they want to know about are workouts and meal plans, thinking this is the first step to finally lose that unwanted body fat. In reality, these are just tools to help reach the final goal. You can't build a house with just a hammer and nails and no blueprint for what it will look like. That might be a pretty funky house if you just grab boards and just starting hammering away!

The same goes with fitness. You need to first visualize what you want to achieve and have the right mindset if you want to succeed. And you can't just visualize it once and be done. Visualization is a continual, daily process and there are many ways to use this powerful strategy to help you reach your full potential and achieve any goal you set your mind to.

So what exactly is visualization? Now I know what you're thinking, this is just some cheesy technique that a lot of the self-help gurus out there talk about and claim that all you need to do is "think positive" and it shall be. This is far from the truth and you can't simply think or wish something into existence like winning the lottery or getting that beach body you've always dreamed of.

Visualization is a well-developed method of improving performance and has been backed by many breakthrough scientific studies and research over the past 20-25 years. Researcher Denis Waitley showed in the 1980's and 1990's, using what he called "Visual Motor Rehearsal" with Olympic Athletes, that when the athletes competed only in their mind, their body showed the same nervous system response comparable to what would occur in the actual event.

Other researchers such as Lynne Evans, Rebecca Haus and Richard Mullen showed that injured athletes and cancer patients demonstrated using visualization techniques to improve rate of healing, increase their ability to deal with the injury or disease, increase motivation to begin doing more on their own, improve their quality of life, decrease their length of hospital stays and also decrease their use of pain medication.

Visualization is a process that involves using all the senses nec-essary to create or recreate an experience in the mind. The key here is using all the senses when applying this technique. You need to really put emotion behind that mental picture in your mind. You need to feel, with as much emotion as you possi-bly can, the experience and believe that you already have your amazing beach body or believe that you have already attained the goals you've set for yourself. This is really powerful and your subconscious mind cannot tell the difference between a mental thought and reality. So eventually, your mind and body will begin to believe what you are visualizing is normal and will seek out ways to help you attract, achieve and maintain what it is you are visualizing.

A good way to practice this is to close your eyes and live in that mental state of already achieving something for a couple min-utes in the morning and the evening. Soon your subconscious will believe this is normal and you'll find ways to attract those goals and successes in your life. I like to use this cool app on iTunes that you could check out called Mind Tuner to help the visualization process and to focus your mind.

The earliest memory I have of using visualization, or mental rehearsal, to help me succeed was back when I was heavily involved in martial arts, specifically Taekwondo, from the age of 8 up until I was about 23. I used visualization in many areas of my martial arts training from testing for a new belt rank to competing in tournaments.

I used a method of visualization I like to call "performance visualization." I didn't really know it at the time nor did I purposely try to use this visualization technique. It was just something that came naturally to me and that I found I habitually did before each rank testing or martial arts competition.

In Taekwondo, once you reach a certain belt rank, you are required to break boards to test your technique and skill level. Visualization really helped me in this area, and board breaking was the most challenging aspect of the rank exam, but at the same time, the most exciting for me. I loved a challenge and I would visualize myself performing each break, my fist or foot, hitting the board dead center and smashing it into two pieces. I would have this vision play over and over again in my head. When it was finally time for me to break my boards, I had already performed it countless times in my head, so my body was ready for the task and gave me the confidence I needed to complete the break.

I also loved competing in tournaments and found I was very successful at it. The night before each competition, I would lie in bed and visualize myself at the tournament. I would see myself throwing perfect punches, kicks and jumps while going through my forms routine. For those who are not familiar, forms are pre-arranged sequences of martial arts techniques, similar to a gymnastics routine, that are performed specific to each belt rank, and increases in difficulty as you achieve a more advanced belt rank or color. I would go through the movements over and over again in my head. I pictured getting perfect scores from the judges, walking up and shaking their hands, as I got handed the first place trophy or medal.

I also visualized the sparring matches and how I would react to punches and kicks being thrown at me and what moves I would use to counter their attack. I had no real idea who my exact competition would be on the day of the tournament, but I visualized an opponent in my head and saw myself winning every time and the judge raising my arm in victory.

So that's how I first discovered visualization and how it helped me. Now that's not to say I broke every board or I won every match, but in my head, I never lost! And that's how you should visualize yourself with whatever you want to achieve. You control the thoughts in your head, so why not make yourself unstoppable.

There are various techniques and ways to use visualization to help you succeed. What I want to focus on in this chapter are three ways you can use it to help you on your journey to becoming more healthy and fit. I use all of these methods with my personal training and boot camp clients to help them continually progress and stay motivated.

The first method is what I call "pre-workout visualization." This is a great technique to get you pumped up for your training session and to get your body ready for a killer workout. To make this the most effective, you should know or have a good idea of the basics of the upcoming workout – like what exercises you'll be doing, how many reps or the time intervals at each station, what equipment you'll be using, etc. Now, say you workout in the morning, as you're getting ready to head out to your training session, see yourself performing each exercise with perfect form and technique. Visualize pushing hard during the workout and challenging yourself to get better on each exercise, maybe doing a harder variation of a lift than before. If you workout in a group class or boot camp, see yourself giving more effort than everybody there, and your workout buddies being amazed at how much energy you're putting into the workout and cheering you on as you complete each set! Trust me, if you start your workout like this, you'll get a much more effective session in, better results and stay safer, because you have already prepared your body for the task at hand. The best part is, all it takes is a couple minutes as you're eating your breakfast or driving to the gym.

Another visualization technique that will help accelerate your fitness results is called "physiological visualization." This is where you try and visualize specific actions taking place in your body – like your muscle fibers getting bigger or the fat burning process happening. One method of physiological visualization that I often use with my clients is to have them imagine specific muscle groups working during each movement pattern. For example, when doing squats, I have them visualize their glute and core muscles engaging and their heels pressing through the floor. To make your imagery as accurate as possible, you could do some research in an anatomy book, but even if you don't know exactly where the muscles are located and what they look like, your body still responds well with the general concept of it and it is still effective.

The final technique I'd like to discuss is called "process visualization." You would use this strategy after you have established your goals. I've used this technique with some of my clients who wanted to lose 2 dress sizes in 60 days or get into their wedding dress in a few short months. Obviously, as the name suggests, you want to mentally see the entire process and not just the final outcome. Sit down and write out your daily action plan needed to achieve the end result. What habits and behaviors do you need to consistently be doing in order to fit into your goal jeans 60 days from now? Then you need to see yourself getting up in the morning and eating a healthy breakfast and going shopping at the store, and filling your cart with lean meats, veggies and fruits. See yourself down at the bar with your friends and only having one drink instead of getting carried away with 5-6 like you normally do, or ordering healthy from the restaurant menu. Visualize getting into the gym consistently every week and really getting in a killer workout each time you're there, instead of just walking on the treadmill while reading the latest issue of Cosmo. Visualize your entire "perfect day" as you want it to unfold, with as much emotion and feeling as possible. This will help prime your brain to carry out those behaviors and habits – so you stay on track to achieve your fitness goals.

Visualization is something that by accident I discovered at a young age, and I'm sure most of you naturally use it too without even realizing it. I've shown you some ways to amplify this simple strategy to help you reach your full potential and by using one or all three of the techniques discussed, you can really accelerate your success and achieve whatever you set your mind to. But just remember this important tip that most people forget to tell you. *Once you have visualized something, you have to take massive action towards the goal you want to achieve.* While visualization has helped me, my clients and can also help you get to your goals faster, <u>taking action is what produces the results</u>.

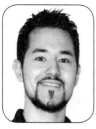

About Mike

Mike Bevard is a certified personal trainer through the American College of Sports Medicine, and has been involved in the fitness industry for over 5 years. Mike is the owner of Capital City Boot Camps and is passionate about helping busy people in the Lincoln area reach their true potential, gain confidence and achieve the bodies they deserve through proper fitness and nutrition.

Mike has also been involved with martial arts for over 15 years and holds a 3rd degree black belt in Taekwondo and 1st degree black belt in Hapkido. He is a two-time world Taekwondo champion and four-time state champion.

To learn more about Mike Bevard or Capital City Boot Camps, visit: www.CapitalCityBootCamps.com and get your free trial to the best boot camp in the Lincoln area.

CHAPTER 9

FIVE STEPS FOR FITNESS SUCCESS

By Daniel Iversen, NASM-CPT, PES

It might be the strangest confession I ever heard.

A friend told me she pays monthly dues at every big gym in town—and she has for years. *Imagine the cost!*

Here's the real kicker, though: she said she never even goes. Amazing, isn't it? Well, later I was thinking about this, and it dawned on me: big gym owners love people like her—especially in January.

Why? Because every January big gyms flood with fresh faces and people waving credit cards. Treadmills grow waiting lines, diet products fly off shelves, and exercise classes burst at the seams.

Unfortunately, every year half of all Americans make New Year's fitness resolutions, but 25 percent give up by the end of the first week. Fifty percent of them fail within six months, and a mere 10 percent stick to their resolutions for an entire year or longer. Yet they keep paying for monthly memberships, plans, and products they never use.

Just like my friend.

Sadly, most people never reach their health and fitness goals. But some succeed and, yes, you can be one of them. You just need to set yourself up for success before you begin. There are five basic steps.

Ready? Let's dig in.

STEP 1: PROGRAM YOUR MENTAL COMPUTER

First, you need to program your mind. When programmed correctly, it steers you toward your goal almost automatically. Careful, though. Given unclear or faulty commands, the mind delivers poor results. That's because negative emotions and old "programs" from your past can cloud your thinking and alter your course.

Think of it this way: imagine a plane on autopilot. Without clear coordinates, the plane will fly out of control, unable to adjust for changes in speed or altitude. That ride won't end well; the plane won't safely reach its destination.

Now, imagine the same airplane with precise coordinates programmed into the flight computer. Adjustments for changes in altitude, wind speed, fuel needs, and other variables will happen almost automatically. That flight will be a pleasant journey, ending in a safe landing.

It sounds strange, but your mind behaves very much like the plane's autopilot computer. Without a clear target, you can't accurately gauge your progress or make adjustments as you move forward. With a clear target, though, you work steadily toward your goal because you know exactly where you are going.

But how do you program your mind? How do you give it a clear target? You program it with pictures, because that's primarily how your mind thinks—and the clearer the picture the better.

So here's what to do: write your fitness goal down; really spell it out. Specify a realistic end date. Use all your senses to create a vivid, detailed picture of your destination—and getting there. In other words, don't write, "I want to lose weight" or, "I vow to lose one hundred pounds in three months!" Instead, write, "I am shedding five pounds of body fat per month for the next six months, for a total of thirty pounds—and I'm fitting into a size-four dress by the Fourth of July. I feel strong, balanced, and energized. I'm smiling in the sun and listening to Johnny Cash as I finish my first 5K. Natural foods taste amazing and I feel nourished."

Next, add to your goal sheet a picture of yourself from when you were thinner and healthier. If you don't have one, find one in a magazine. This is what your goal looks like. Some people create "goal boards" or "dream boards," where they paste several pictures and words related to their goals. Make one of these and hang it up where you can see it every day. Getting this repeated visual reminder has a powerful effect on your brain.

To make sure you stay on target, mark your calendar with monthly checkpoints. To accurately judge your progress and make appropriate adjustments, have a certified personal trainer record your body fat, weight, and circumference measurements. Or, purchase a kit and learn to do it yourself.

These measurements and recorded goal statements give you a jumping-off point and a clear target. *Without them, you're flying blind.*

Now deepen your success programming with Step Two.

STEP 2: DISCOVER *WHY* YOU WANT YOUR GOAL

Once you know your target, you can start your journey. To really travel swiftly, however, you need high-octane "mental fuel."

What creates high-octane mental fuel? Pain. You need to discover the true, painful reason you want to take action. Why? Because we rarely take action until we feel pain or feel threatened with pain. Pain is your deepest reason for wanting change, and this ultimate emotional "why" behind your goal is your fuel.

Often the pain hides itself behind superficial goals. You'll have to do some digging.

Here's how: read your goal out loud, and then ask yourself *why* you want it. When you get an answer, follow that with another "why?" Keep going until it feels uncomfortable—and personal. Remember, this is about *you*. Getting to the bottom of your reasons will help you tap into your most powerful motivation.

Your inner dialogue might go something like this: "I want to fit into smaller clothes again. Why? So I won't feel like such a blob. Why does that matter to me? Because I feel like people aren't seeing the real me, the attractive me. This makes me feel trapped. Why is that so bad?"

And so on. Keep questioning yourself until you run out of answers…

Here's another one: "I want to be fit and have more energy. Why? Because I don't like being winded after climbing a flight of stairs or chasing my kids. Why? Because it's embarrassing and I feel guilty for letting myself go. And it makes me feel old, which I hate. I want to feel young again… I want to be around for a long, long time!"

Only when you have peeled back all the layers will you arrive at the real emotional reason behind your desire for change. It's pain, but it's also your high-octane fuel.

Now you have another crucial step.

STEP 3: DETERMINE THE COST

Your goal comes at a price. You'll have to pay through EFFORT, SELF-DISCIPLINE, and PERSONAL RESPONSIBILITY. The costs may also include sacrifice: eliminating junk food, giving up cocktail hour with friends, devoting free time to daily exercise, for example. You may have to say good-bye to enablers who don't have your best interests in mind. Also, if you don't know the physical steps to reach your fitness goal, it may cost the price of a competent trainer or coach.

Figure out the total cost of achieving your goal and write it down. You need to get it out of your head—where it's vague and negotiable—and onto paper—where it's concrete and fixed. Writing down the cost also helps to eliminate surprises, which can derail you along the way. Just as it's important to identify the motivating pain behind your goal in Step 2, it's critical to specify the actual cost of getting there.

After you determine what you will have to pay to achieve your goal, then it's time do what most won't.

STEP 4: TAKE ACTION

All of the preceding steps help—tremendously. But unless you are willing to take action, nothing will happen.

Are you willing to take action? If you are, be aware of some simple but important actions that others often avoid (or fail to do):

- Keeping a food journal to track workouts and food intake
- Showing up for every workout
- Giving up unhealthy foods and drinks
- Hiring expert help for guidance, encouragement, and accountability
- Following a proven food plan instead of trying fad diets
- Committing to a plan instead of just "winging it"
- Setting a date and following through

If you aren't willing to pay the price of getting somewhere, your journey will end abruptly.

So take action: Set your goals, get a plan, get started, and follow through. Think of that old adage: a journey of a thousand miles begins with a single step. Take it.

Now let's take the last step to clear away remaining obstacles.

STEP 5: MENTAL HOUSEKEEPING

I had a client once who decided to give up before she even started. She couldn't see the point of trying when she knew she would only fail in the end. After all, she had failed before.

After some digging, she realized it was all just a failure fantasy, a sort of learned helplessness. She had trapped herself in a negative picture generated solely by fear, not based on reality.

If we believe we will fail, failure is our destiny.

To change her destiny, my client changed her beliefs. She generated a success fantasy by focusing on her goal statements and dream board daily. She saw herself succeeding in her mind's eye, reading her goals aloud every morning, deeply experiencing the feeling of achieving her goal, and focusing only on what she wanted—never on the possibility of failure. She mentally rehearsed her success over and over. Eventually her mind "flipped" and she felt like putting in the effort, because she decided she was going to succeed.

Here are her results so far:

- She has lost fifty-nine pounds (…and still counting)
- She left a toxic relationship because the stress was causing her to overeat
- She looks, feels, and acts about ten years younger
- Her clothes look *HOT* on her (her words)
- People notice her and she inspires them to get in shape

She's a changed person.

Do this: take a deep breath, close your eyes, and dream about how you WANT to look and feel… Get clear about what you really want, visualize and *feel* what it would be like to get it. Do this every time you read your goal statements. The repetition will help reprogram your mind for success.

If, like my transformed friend above, you find yourself obsessing over imagined failures in the future... or if you constantly think, What if this goes wrong?... or, What if I blow it? Then you are creating your own personal horror film—which is a big problem, because the nervous system can't tell the difference between a real and vividly imagined event.

Think about the last time you were deeply absorbed in a movie. If it was a tearjerker, maybe you cried. But the movie was only a fantasy. Nothing *actually* went wrong. It was just your nervous system responding to those vividly imagined scenarios. It was *as if* they were real.

Einstein said, "Imagination is everything. It is the preview of life's coming attractions." Why not imagine the future the way you want it to be? The fact is, every passing moment is another opportunity to turn it all around.

YOU CAN SUCCEED—IF YOU TAKE ACTION

The five steps described above are simple enough. But they only work if you are willing to actually follow through and take them. You have to make a decision. That's the ultimate key.

Get started today. Find a quiet space. Imagine your body, your health, and your life exactly as you wish them to be. Focus on your goal and the solutions. Get out your pen, and then:

1. Create a crystal-clear goal to program your mind.
2. Determine WHY you want the goal.
3. Determine the actions and tools you need to get there—the price you must pay.
4. Decide if you are willing to take action, and then do it.
5. Clear away mental obstacles with new beliefs about yourself and your abilities.

The most important tool in your self-transformational arsenal is your mind. You must overcome doubt and take action.

Nothing happens until you begin. So get started now. Take action.

Yes, you can!

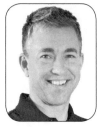

About Daniel

Daniel Iversen spends his waking hours helping people reach their fitness and personal goals faster. Since 1996, he has literally taught thousands of men and women how to take control of their minds and bodies; to embrace health, and seize the ever-present opportunity to improve. For three years, he had the top radio show in Portland called *"The Noon-Workout"* where he took live calls. Every month he shares fitness secrets on Portland's morning show: AM Northwest, and has been featured in *USA Today, The Oregonian, The Herald-Leader, Portland Monthly,* as well as Fox and ABC affiliate stations.

If you live in Portland, Oregon, you can work with Daniel at Portland Adventure Boot Camp for Women where he's helped women of all shapes, sizes, and lifestyles get the body and health they really want – since 2006.

To learn more about Daniel Iversen, and get mountains of free self-help information, go to: www.PortlandBootCamp.com
Email: Daniel@Portlandbootcamp.com
Or call: 503-946-8709

CHAPTER 10

"METABOLIC TYPING" AND OTHER DIETARY APPROACHES

– Why Everyone Is Right and Wrong
At the Same Time, PLUS
– 3 Diet Steps YOU Can Take To Make
YOU Bigger, Better, Faster, Stronger!

By Eirith Garza

My journey learning about food began not through any formal education, but in high school when I unnecessarily bulked (fattened) up to an unfavorable 220 lb. and over 30% bodyfat in an attempt to get bigger, better, faster, and stronger for sports. Always being the smaller guy, I felt that I deserved to be bigger and better, and if having a gut (which didn't seem that big of a deal to me) was required, then so be it. I put on about 80 lb. of mass (most which I know was fat) in 6 months. This was done through uncontrolled eating at many times of the day. I ingested much unhealthy food like muffins or bags of Potato Chips to obtain mass. I succeeded and actually became much stronger.

I started out a puny 139 lb. at 5'6, and then ballooned to 220. At this point I knew I had taken it too far, and one day of sitting on a couch watching TV, a sharp pain went down my left arm* caused me to start actually "dieting" and my journey to understand the human body's interaction with nutrients.

I went on a cyclical ketogenic diet and lost a considerable amount of weight by my graduation six months later. Going from a blubbery 220 to a slightly pudgy 186, I maintained and even gained strength. I continued on this diet for years attempting to find that elusive six-pack. I did, but not without losing hard-earned muscle mass. As I continued on this plan for even longer (I started it in 2004 and continued on to 2007 off and on), I saw very little progress, and I noticed I got considerably weaker. Ironically, this is when my personal training career began. I had learned more about how nutrition interacts with the human body than the many years working out "training" myself. My clients pushed me to become better at mastering nutrition because any lack of progress on their part would hinder me professionally.

Around the time I started studying nutrition, I was finishing up my fitness study program. Around this time I was satisfied with my fat-loss progress and I was ready to try and put on muscle mass again. At this time, I was introduced to John Berardi's articles. Being an avid fan of the notorious Testosterone Magazine and T-Nation, I took the advice. Among the advice included different dietary approaches to adding muscle, which included high carb, moderate carb, and low carb approaches. Berardi concluded that depending on an individual's insulin sensitivity (how well they uptake glucose in their body), different diets may be prescribed to avoid fat gain when trying to ADD weight. The pancreas produces insulin to regulate blood sugar, and how much insulin you produce determines insulin sensitivity. Low production signals high sensitivity (and high hunger control), and high production signals insulin insensitivity and low hunger control. High carb diets were prescribed for people with great insulin sensitivity, moderate carbs for moderate insulin sensitivity, and low carbs for poor insulin sensitivity. The better the "sensitivity," the more carbs one could eat. I read that ketogenic diets wrecked insulin sensitivity, so I panicked.

Desperate to know that I could eat carbs, I began to research many books and resources on insulin sensitivity. My journey took me into understanding what is necessary to gain muscle and lose fat effectively. I came to understand dietary dogma as merely that, and saw that objective approaches to the ideal body, rather than a one-size-fits-all strategy. Here I did verify Berardi's teachings for myself, all while learning through self-experimentation.

When I first began learning about how different sensitivities affect leanness, I decided to start with a low carb approach. As is a common practice for bodybuilders to slowly re-introduce carbs into their body after a low carb diet, I followed, knowing that my insulin sensitivity was probably lowered. What happened was a drawn-out period of adding one piece of fruit per week for 20 weeks until I had reached a moderate carb intake. Around this time, I started working at a new gym, and I noticed all of the other trainers were much larger and leaner than me. I needed to understand nutrition or else I felt my credibility as a trainer would suffer. I compiled a list of resources and came up with some guidelines as to how this can be applied.

Generally, as Berardi said, it is accurate to say that not one approach fits everyone. Anyone who believes that their diet is superior is either a layperson with little experience, a quack with specific products to sell, or some brainwashed cult-follower against whom research and alternate theories are useless. Interestingly enough, I've been in some form of those three stages at some point, but research caused me to oppose the dogma. Because not one diet is superior, it is imperative to know your individual insulin sensitivity if you want the diet to work for you. The research I found corroborated with Berardi's, especially one interesting study that found superior fat loss based on insulin sensitivity and different diet plans. Obese women of different insulin sensitivities were prescribed different diets, and those with corresponding sensitivities according to the diet lost the most weight, and vice versa [1]. So while it's possible for everyone to lose weight, the type of diet will determine how effective the diet will be for weight loss [2]. Now, when I say diet, keep in mind I am referring to a set of guidelines based on specific levels of macronutrients, not any sort of "eat this, not that" nonsense. The Laws of Thermodynamics do not change the caloric density of a food, and contrary to what people think, eating "dirty" is not a deterrent to weight loss or even to favorable body composition [3,4]. But, once you do know your insulin sensitivity, you can do the diet that fits you. How do you find a diet that fits you? There are 3 simple steps:

1) Determine your blood sugar levels

2) Find your nutrient type

3) Set up your diet

Step 1) Determine Blood Sugar Levels

So how do you find out your insulin sensitivity? A simple doctor's visit does the trick. Getting your blood sugar checked in a fasted state will let you know. If you fall within an 80-100 range in fasted blood glucose, your insulin sensitivity is moderate and moderate carb and fat intakes are best. If your blood glucose reads above 100, your insulin sensitivity is poor and low carbs are best. If your blood glucose reads below 80, your insulin sensitivity is good and higher carbs and best. But what if for some reason you can't obtain tests like these? Heard of Metabolic Typing?

Step 2) Find Your Nutrient Type

A test on "Metabolic Typing" exists in which many external factors are measured to determine whether you are a "protein" or "carbo" type. It takes into account aspects of a person's body chemistry such as whether they feel colder, have dry skin, or whether they feel energized when they eat foods like meat. This test is simply a questionnaire and is subjective, as your own taste for foods or how cold you feel may/may not affect your individual blood sugar. Those who have read mainstream books may have seen variations of this questionnaire. The problem here is that it is incredibly easy to misinterpret. Unless you go to a doctor and get your blood sugar (fasted) levels checked, you won't have a definitive answer. A better subjective test would be to simply examine which type of diet gets you leaner or fatter. If you find that carbs tire you out, make you sluggish and just make you experience energy swings and crashes, you'd do well on a low carb diet. If you find your energy stable and can function well with carbs, use a higher carb diet [1]. Research has shown however that there are high and low fat phenotypes [5], which simply means people who handle high dietary fat intakes do either poorly or well. Another study also shows how varying levels of carb intake affected weight loss depending on individual insulin sensitivity [6]. So while there is validity to such questionnaires, they are still very subjective.

Step 3)   Set Up Your Diet
If you seek something objective, pay for the blood test. If your levels are within 80-100 mg/dl, your insulin sensitivity is moderate, meaning you can do well on an "isocaloric" diet that breaks down all calories evenly, such as a 33/33/33 (percentages) diet comprised of 33% protein, 33% carbs, and 33% fat. Barry Sears popularized isocaloric diets with The Zone, a 30/40/30 diet (protein/carbs/fat). Some bodybuilders prefer a 40% protein diet and the other 30% carbs and 30% fat. If your insulin sensitivity is on the lower end of the moderate region (aka 90-100), you can go with a 40% Fat, 30% Protein, 30% Carb diet. The reason this is the case is because fat has the least impact on insulin levels, and the more controlled carbs are, the higher fat goes. Generally, protein cannot be set VERY high for insulin resistant individuals, as too much protein raises insulin, too. This is why many low carb diets are high in fat. Generally, fat increases when carbs decrease, and protein should be set high regardless, so protein needs tend to stay constant. A good rule of thumb is 30-35% of caloric level for all approaches.

If your score is above 100, then you have insulin resistance (slight if below 110, and pre-diabetic if above 110). Low carb, high fat diets would work best in this case. Many people who "fail" with traditional low fat diets find higher fat, low carb diets to work wonders for them. A low carb diet is to be understood as a diet wherein carbs make up less than $1/3^{rd}$ of the calories, so a diet that is 25% carbs is low. Extreme low carb diets drop carbs below 100 grams a day, and these are the ketogenic diets I spoke of earlier.

One of my clients went on one after his wife adopted the lifestyle. They both noticed the plan aided their health. Two other clients, one a 46-year-old male who had started at 35% bodyfat, the other a 28-year-old female who started at around 38% bodyfat, found much success as well. Energy levels skyrocketed, health improved, lipids stabilized, and blood pressure dropped. These people provide anecdotal evidence for the effectiveness of low carbing. However, another client, a 56-year-old female with similar stats to the others did absolutely terrible on it. When she switched to an isocaloric diet, the pounds started coming off. Of course, some degree of adherence to the diet (isocaloric diets are easier to adhere to than low carb diets) might have played a role. Her body chemistry might have not been ideal for that approach. I personally FAILED MISERABLY on a low carb diet, losing only lean muscle and stalling at a mediocre body fat level. Since switching to a high carb, low fat approach, I actually managed to get to single digit bodyfat. This brings me to the final option in different diet plans, the low-fat, high-carb option.

However, this option does NOT work for most people. As most people do not have enough physical activity in their lives and some degree of insulin resistance, this diet is what causes many a failure. However, since you are reading this book, we can assume you have some amount of physical activity in your life. All you need to know is whether your score is above 80 or not. So what constitutes low fat, anyway? For some, low fat means skinning their chicken, buying tuna in water, and eating brown rice and broccoli, leaving trace fat. For practical purposes, we'll assume low fat is anything less than 1/3rd of your calories (just based off percentages), so if someone eats 25% fat, this is a "low" fat diet. "High" carb simply means high in relation to the other nutrients, so it is subjective. A high carb, low fat diet can be 45% Carbs, 30% Protein, and 25% Fat. As far as calories are concerned, a good resource is: www.calorieking.com to track your calories and see how many you might need.

So let's summarize the above in *The 3 Steps To A Better Diet*:

1. Determine your blood sugar levels: If you fall between 80-100, you have moderate insulin sensitivity; below 80 is good insulin sensitivity, and above 100 is poor insulin sensitivity.

2. Find your nutrient type: Moderate insulin sensitivity will require a moderate carb/fat diet, good insulin sensitivity will require a high carb, low fat diet, and poor insulin sensitivity will require a low carb diet.

3. Set up your diet!: Pick foods that are either moderate, high, or low in carbs and fat so as to fit your daily caloric needs.

Those are the 3 steps to a better diet. It's really that simple. There is no right answer in what type of diet is best; it's all about YOU and how YOUR body is. So if you find yourself merely spinning your wheels and not finding any results (or not getting the results you want) with your current eating program, simply go ahead and apply the above steps and watch your body change.

Do this and you too will be bigger, better, faster, and stronger!

REFERENCES

1. Cornier MA et al. *Insulin sensitivity determines the effectiveness of dietary macronutrient composition on weight loss in obese women.* Obes Res. 2005 Apr;13(4):703-9.

2. Pittas AG, Roberts SB. *Dietary composition and weight loss: can we individualize dietary prescriptions according to insulin sensitivity or secretion status?* Nutr Rev. 2006 Oct;64(10 Pt 1):435-48. Review.

3. Madero M, et al. *The effect of two energy-restricted diets, a low-fructose diet versus a moderate natural fructose diet, on weight loss and metabolic syndrome parameters: a randomized controlled trial.* Metabolism. 2011 May 27. [Epub ahead of print.]

4. Surwit RS, et al. M*etabolic and behavioral effects of a high-sucrose diet during weight loss.* Am J Clin Nutr. 1997 Apr;65(4):908-15.

5. Blundell JE, Cooling J. *High-fat and low-fat (behavioral) phenotypes: biology or environment?* Proc Nutr Soc. 1999 Nov;58(4):773-7.

6. Pittas AG et. al. *A low-glycemic load diet facilitates greater weight loss in overweight adults with high insulin secretion but not in overweight adults with low insulin secretion in the CALERIE Trial. Diabetes* Care. 2005 Dec;28(12):2939-41.

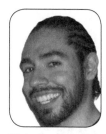

About Eirith

Name: Eirith Garza

City: Chicago, IL

Company: Chicagoland Fitness Camp

Website: http://skokiepersonaltrainer.com
http://northshoreweightloss.com, and
http://fb.com/SkokieBootCamp

Work Phone: (847)790-4FIT

List of Education, Honors and Awards

University/College/Certifications:

Robert Morris University: Associate of Applied Science in Fitness and Exercise
Elmhurst College: Pursuing Bachelor's of Science in Exercise Science
National Personal Training Institute: Nutrition and Personal Trainer Certifications
American Council of Exercise: Certified Personal Trainer

Honors:

LA Fitness: Personal Training Star (given to trainers with the most PT clients), King Of The Hill (same as previous, but highest level), and #1 on Personal Trainer Leaderboard (given to trainers w/most clients with best results.)

Media:

Eirith Garza and Chicagoland Fitness Camp featured in *Crain's Chicago Business*

CHAPTER 11

How to Become a Fat-Buring Machine Without Losing Muscle.

By Carlos Arias

CARBOHYDRATE CONUNDRUM

The American public is under the impression that carbohydrates are the main source of fuel for their daily activities. They believe that without glucose, the brain cannot function. We've been programmed to believe this through misleading marketing and loose science. I remember learning about the Food Pyramid when I was in elementary school. At the base, the USDA recommended an arbitrary 6-11 servings of bread, pasta, cereal and rice per day. That is over a cup of sugar a day, well over the recommended 5 grams of sugar the body needs for optimal function. Look around and you'll find a plump population that has reduced their fat intake, yet their waistlines continue to grow.

LIPID HYPOTHESIS

The lipid hypothesis is the idea that cholesterol causes heart disease.

In simple terms, the lipid hypothesis is as follows:

1) cholesterol and/or fat in the blood causes plaque formation in the arteries and, consequently, heart disease.

2) cholesterol and/or fat in the diet leads to cholesterol and/or fat in the blood; and, therefore...

3) cholesterol and/or fat in the diet causes heart disease.

In 1953, Dr. Ancel Keys introduced the hypothesis that consumption of fat raises blood cholesterol, which in turn causes death from heart disease. The notion that fat causes heart disease eventually became known as the lipid hypothesis and gave birth to catch phrases such as "artery-clogging saturated fats". Sounds simple enough, but the problem is that there is no hard science behind it. One scientifically-verified fact disproves the myth altogether: only about half the people who have heart attacks have elevated cholesterol levels.

PALEOLITHIC DIET

By now, it is well known that humans evolved eating meat, seafood, vegetables, fruits and nuts. Our starches came primarily from roots and tubers (think sweet potatoes and yucca). Plantains are also on the list of approved starches. In essence, you want to avoid grains, legumes and dairy. So that means no rice, pasta, bread, most beans, milk, cheese and yogurts. This is contrary to the "norm" but then again, we are only getting sicker as a population. Avoid these items like you would anything that makes you sick. Although you obviously would want to strive for 100%, just do the best you can. Google "Paleo Diet" and you'll find thousands of mouth-watering recipes. Read the literature and try it for yourself. I have no doubt that it will leave a positive impact on the quality of your life as it has done for myself, my family and my most dedicated clients.

FAT FOR FUEL

Paleolithic man didn't have food readily available every three hours. He didn't eat 5-6 small meals a day. In fact, sometimes he would go hours, if not days without eating. Needless to say, caveman carbohydrate consumption was negligible at best. In the absence of Carbohydrates the body turns to fat for fuel. Most people believe that glucose is the primary fuel source of the body. These people fall in two categories: they're either genetically gifted (a mere 5-10% of the population) or have a soft body type ("skinny-fat" or "just-fat"). They are the same ones that always avoid dietary fat and reach for whole-wheat grains to get their fiber. Lucky for you, I am here to tell you otherwise.

KETOGENIC DIET

A ketogenic diet is a high-fat, low-carbohydrate, adequate-protein diet that was intended primarily to treat epilepsy in children. The diet forces the body to burn fats rather than carbohydrates. This means that the body will start breaking down your own body fat to fuel the body's normal, every day functions and activities. Americans seldom reach ketosis, since we slam our metabolic-engine with far too many carbohydrates. When your body has been completely depleted of carbohydrates (glucose), the pancreas releases Ketone Bodies in response. A KB is manufactured in the liver through the Krebs cycle. When the body has no glycogen to run off of, the pancreas will then release the hormone glucagon. Glucagon is a catabolic hormone, meaning it will break down your body tissues for energy. For our intended purposes, glucagon is highly important, since it helps convert free fatty acids into ketones. The ketones can be used by your cells in place of the missing sugars, thanks to the body's ability to switch its metabolic engine on the go.

In other words, since you've burned up all your stored glycogen (carbohydrates), and you don't have any new food coming in, ketosis kicks in, and your body uses the fat that was stored from a previous meal (or on your waist) to fuel itself. Consider the fact that only small amounts of glucose can be stored as glycogen for fuel. What would have happened to all Paleolithic humans if they didn't have ketones to burn when we couldn't find any food for a week? Our hunter-gatherer ancestors would have run out of stored sugar by lunch, and not had any energy to run down their dinner. In fact, researchers have discovered that the body and brain actually prefer to burn ketone bodies over glucose.

The state of ketosis is for the most part controlled by insulin, glucagon, and blood glucose levels. Insulin is a hormone that is secreted by the pancreas in the presence of carbohydrates. Insulin's purpose is to keep blood glucose levels balanced by acting as a driver, delivering the glucose to the blood. If insulin were not to be secreted, blood glucose levels would get out of control and have deleterious effects on the body.

Glucagon on the other hand, is insulin's antagonistic hormone, which is also secreted by the pancreas. When a person skips meals or does not consume adequate amounts of carbohydrates for an extended period of time, Insulin levels drop. Glucagon is secreted by the pancreas to signal the break down of the body's glycogen stores. But what happens if this continues and liver glycogen runs out? This is where the metabolic state of ketosis kicks in. Ketosis is when the pancreas begins breaking down free fatty acids into a usable energy substrate, also known as ketones, or ketone bodies. Simply put, you'll be burning body-fat faster for fuel, and dropping pounds faster than ever before.

MUSCLE-SPARING

What makes the Ketogenic Diet special is its ability to spare muscle while burning fat for fuel. Always remember that muscle mass is gold! It costs much time, effort and money to build an ounce of functional muscle, so do what you must to keep it. Many popular diets are low-carb, but they don't discriminate between muscle and fat. If you are trying to "lose weight" it is important to hold on to as much muscle as possible, so as to keep your metabolism operating at an optimal level. You'll need around 0.75g of protein per pound of lean body mass and 1 to 1.25g of fat per pound. You find your LBM by subtracting your body fat from your overall bodyweight. So, if you're a male that weighs 200 pounds at 10 percent bodyfat, you carry 20 pounds of fat and your lean body mass is 180 pounds. If you are trying to gain muscle and burn fat, eat 1.5g of fat per pound, and 1g of protein per pound throughout the whole day. It is okay to reach for whey protein powders in order to reach your daily goals.

StrongerFasterHealthier.com offers Grass-Fed Protein Powder, which is "Paleo-Friendly" and tastes fantastic! I recommend 1 or 2 scoops of protein, one-third can of coconut milk, 2-3 ice cubes and a handful of berries. It's the healthiest smoothie you'll find anywhere. As far as daily calories are concerned: If you are trying to gain weight you'll need 20+ calories per pound of bodyweight. To maintain your weight, you are looking at 15-17 calories per pound and to lose weight, you'll need 12-15 calories per pound of bodyweight.

INTERMITTENT FASTING (IF)

Unless you are raiding the refrigerator several times throughout the night, you are doing some form of IF. When you sleep, you have intermittently fasted throughout the night. So if you slept eight hours, you just had an 8 hour fast. Some people fast 12-hours, while others go a full 24-hrs, also known as "fast & feast." Our Paleolithic ancestors did not have groceries lining their cave shelves. Hell, they didn't even have shelves, let alone 5-6 small meals a day, spread out evenly over 2-3 hours. This has been the personal trainer mantra for over a decade now and I am just sick of hearing it. Unless you are a highly active athlete, or trying to gain weight, you don't need to be eating exactly every 3 hours. You would be better off eating in certain windows throughout your day. You can use your sleep time as your "baseline" fast.

From there, I recommend the following approach. On day one, fast for 10 hours including the time you slept (8+2=10). The next day, add an hour, so 11 hours. The third day will demand 12 hours, and so on. Continue this for 6 days (Mon-Sat), and incrementally, you'll reach 15 hours with barely any pain. On day 7, implement Re-Feed Strategy (explained below) and start again at 10 hours on Monday to repeat the process. This can go on all year round. The science on this is new, but many people are having phenomenal results with I.F.

Be sure to have a strategy in place to meet your daily caloric needs based on your goals. Also, during your fast, you cannot eat or drink anything but water, tea or black coffee. No sugar and definitely no artificial sweeteners. If you are trying to gain or maintain weight, I.F. is not for you.

RE-FEED STRATEGY

Increase your carbohydrates and limit your fat intake on your toughest training days (sprinting, heavy lifting, high intensity workouts or anything that results in glycogen depletion). But don't cut Fat out altogether, simply emphasize carbs over fat, but keep them around 100g-120g of carbohydrates either on Saturday or Sunday. Keep your protein the same at 1g of protein per lean body mass. Limit your re-feeds to once a week if you have round features, and twice a week if you have more "square angles" in your physique. Avoid grains and beans and go for cleaner carbohydrate choices: sweet potatoes, plantains, squash, yams and limited fruit (one fruit per day max). Lastly, finish your carb re-feed with a high protein meal.

PUTTING IT ALL TOGETHER

The layering and timing will be of utmost importance. It'll ensure you are getting the most burning of fat while preserving precious muscle tissue. I recommend the following:

Monday through Saturday: implement both the Ketogenic Diet and Intermittent Fasting. It will require some written organization on your part, but what gets written down, gets done.

On Saturday evening, begin your "Re-Feed" by including significant amounts of carbohydrates at every meal from "Paleo-

Approved" sources such as yams and sweet potatoes. Continue this throughout your weekend, while still adhering to the Intermittent Fasting Schedule. Sunday evening, eat a high protein meal, and begin Monday with the Ketogenic Diet. At some point you will reach 15 hours of fasting, just start again with your sleep time plus two hours as your "base" fast, and continue to incrementally add an hour everyday to your fast. Like all effective diet programs, this one will require a logbook.

WHAT TO EXPECT?

One of the main benefits of a Ketogenic Diet is that it increases the body's ability to utilize your fats for fuel. This ability is normally drowned out by the constant hammering of carbohydrates by the American diet. Also, Ketosis has a muscle-sparing effect when you eat adequate amounts of protein in relation to your size. The last benefit that I'll point out, is that a Ketogenic Diet has a way of blunting your hunger as time progresses. Appetite loss is a great ally to have while fighting body-fat.

Nothing in life is without its drawbacks. The first few weeks of this diet will provide you with a feeling of lethargy. You'll feel a mental fog as your metabolism switches fuels from glucose to ketones. This metabolic shift is necessary, so stick to the program and tough it out. Another drawback is that due to the limited amounts of carbohydrates one consumes, micronutrient deficiencies can occur. To steer clear from this, eat tons of greens, good fats and supplement with multivitamins and even BCAAs. The last drawback is the potential state of ketoacidosis, which occurs when the level of ketones reaches a dangerous level. But this is not a concern for us, since we are not going weeks at a time in Ketosis, but instead, a mere five and a half days before we re-feed with clean carbohydrates.

PHYSICAL TRAINING PROTOCOL

The general population is absolutely obsessed with "high-intensity" anything. I guess it is because people link the burning sensation in muscles to the burning of body fat. This, of course, is absolutely wrong. A sprinter and a marathoner use different sources of fuel. If you are overweight, you want to limit your high-intensity work to once or twice a week. Workouts that are of high-intensity deplete your glycogen stores (great for Monday, after Re-Feed), but if you go too far, it will only make you hungrier and ultimately fatter.

Most of your physical training efforts should be directed towards a solid practical and prudent functional strength-training program. Low to moderate intensity exercise works wonders for the overweight and overstressed. Needless to say, nothing beats gets getting a Coach or a Trainer. I'd recommend finding a "Strength-Biased" CrossFit gym in your area that teaches small classes so as to avoid getting "lost in the sauce." Do your research, since the quality of training varies (and is largely unregulated) between CrossFit affiliates.

Most always choose compound movements (multi-joint, i.e. squat, bench press, etc.) over isolation movements for maximum effectiveness. They are superior in darn near every way. The benefits of being strong cannot be overstated and compound movements get you there.

In all training scenarios, it needs to be said that recovery is key. It is during your recovery periods that you will make your gains, not during your training efforts. So rest and rest well. We're talking a sleep time of 8-9 hours in a pitch-black room, adequate water, plenty of sun and a happy state of mind. This, I believe, is the key to reaching your goals and more importantly, keeping them for life.

Eat Clean, Train Hard & Sleep Well.

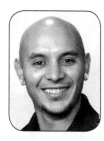

About Carlos

Carlos Arias, also known as "The Nutrition Guy," is a Strength and Nutrition practitioner and expert. Carlos is an Operation Iraqi Freedom Veteran and a former member of the elite U.S. Marine Corps Special Operations Command.

Carlos is a Head Coach and Owner of Animus CrossFit in Miami Gardens, Florida. He is currently pursuing a Bachelor's Degree in Exercise Physiology at Barry University.

Carlos can be reached at: Carlos@AnimusCrossFit.com or at (305) 653-3838.

CHAPTER 12

The Top Seven Nutritional Supplements You Need to Know About

By Philip Cook

It's awfully hard to be Bigger, Better, Faster, Stronger if you neglect the nutritional side of the formula. As the owner of multiple nutrition stores in the Raleigh, NC market, I have had the opportunity to work with thousands of customers and athletes and to hear the feedback of what works and what does not work in the area of nutritional supplements. In this chapter you will see my current top 7 picks of 'must have' supplements for those in search of a Bigger, Better, Faster, Stronger body.

For many of us, it's a leap of faith to take supplements in the hope that they may provide a benefit....down the road. Overall, I firmly believe that the science and studies bear out that supplementation with the right product can improve your health. I have been taking supplements and studying them since my college days at NC State University. I remember one of my first reactions to Vitamin B3, known as niacin. I found it in the kitchen cabinet where my dad kept his vitamins. Somewhere I read that niacin might be effective in helping maintain good cholesterol levels. So I figured that if taking one tablet would be helpful why not take three? Well I found out why you should not take three high dose niacin tablets about twenty minutes later when my neck and ears started burning like they were on fire! I was having a niacin flush. So as you read through my top picks below, remember that more is not always better.

1. MULTI-VITAMIN DRINK

I'm sure you saw this one coming. Take a really good multi-vitamin every day. Why? Because the typical American diet is one of the worst in the world. Our food intake has become devoid of nutrients and antioxidants that come from fruits and vegetables. We now live in the land of drive-thru windows and processed foods. Our parents mostly ate better than we do now and their parents ate even better. While growing up in Hickory, NC my father always had a garden, grape vines, strawberries, and fruit trees. For a few years we even had two gardens to tend to, so we had a lot of fresh vegetables. We had so many that my mom canned a lot of vegetables. Now, we are all too busy to grow our own food.

Why do you think the American Cancer Society recommends the consumption of 5-7 servings of fresh fruits and vegetables every day? It's the protective effect that the antioxidants, nutrients, and fiber can potentially have on your body. Now, I am certainly not saying that a vitamin supplement can replace food, but it can ensure that you are getting a close equivalent base of nutrients that many Americans lack.

Notice I recommend that you take a powdered multi-vitamin that is mixed into your own good clean water. This will provide a liquid method of consumption far superior to pills or tablets. There have been many studies done, and the resounding answer is that the advantages of consuming a liquid-based vitamin far outweighs pill-based products. One of the most referred-to statements is found in the Physician's Desk Reference. In this widely used medical reference book, it is noted that liquids can be absorbed up to 98%. Whereas it states the absorption rate of pills and capsules is 5% - 18%.

Other advantages of a liquid multi-vitamin are:

- Fewer doses required to receive the same amount absorbed into the body
- Liquids are far simpler to swallow, particularly for seniors
- Liquid ingredients are not compressed, which would require additional digestion by the human body before assimilation into the bloodstream
- Unlike pills, liquids do not require any sort of buffers, binders or fillers, which would (again) cause an additional delay in digestion – in other words, taking more time to enter the bloodstream

Try to find a powdered multi-vitamin that also includes a base of phytonutrients. These plant-based micronutrients are sorely lacking in most daily meals. One product I recommend is the Nature's Fuel™ powdered multi-vitamin. This product is available at your local Nutrishop™ retailer.

2. MOLECULARLY DISTILLED FISH OIL

There have been multiple studies over the years that lend evidence that the supplementation of fish oil or consumption of fresh cold water fish can provide a host of benefits. Most Americans do not consume 2-3 servings of fresh fish per week thereby are lacking in the intake of the Omega-3 fatty acids. By taking docosahexaenoic acid (DHA) and eicosapentaenoic acid (EPA) in the form of fish oil supplements you may experience lower triglycerides, lower the risk of heart attack and dangerous abnormal heart rhythms, lessen the risk of stroke in people with known cardiovascular disease, slow the buildup of atherosclerotic plaques ("hardening of the arteries"), and lower blood pressure slightly.

A recommended dose of fish oil is usually in the range of 1-3 grams per day. I recommend to my customers that they take a product that is molecularly distilled. A molecular distillation process takes the fish and removes the toxins and other contaminants in our environment, such as heavy metals like mercury and other metals along with PCBs.

3. VITAMIN D

With all of the recommendations over the past decade to use sun screen and limit your exposure to direct sun light, the importance of Vitamin D has ever-growing evidence supporting supplementation. This fat-soluble vitamin can be found in small amounts in a few foods such as sardines and mackerel. Vitamin D is can also be synthesized from sun exposure or obtained in supplement form.

Vitamin D is essential for the efficient utilization of calcium by the body which leads to bone health and density. Other research is now showing links to other benefits such as enhancing immune system function, reducing the risk of colorectal cancer.

I don't know if being a lifeguard over several summers caused it, but I have had several skin cancer cells removed, thus limiting my exposure to a lot of sun. So supplementation is important, plus I just don't eat as many sardines as I used to. Currently, the Institute of Medicine (IOM) has set the Recommended Daily Allowance for Vitamin D at 600IUs. Recently the IOM has upped the safer tolerable limit from 2000IUs to 4000IUs. The most popular dose sold in my store currently is the 5000IUs.

4. ARGININE

Many of the customers that come into my nutrition stores think that Arginine is strictly a bodybuilding supplement, and that's just not the case. It's so much more because of what it does. This amino acid helps your body create more nitric oxide.

Nitric oxide helps keep arteries relaxed and pliable for normal blood pressure and allows for greater circulation. In the gym, guys talk about a greater pump. This "pump" effect is the engorgement of muscle fiber with oxygen rich blood and is delivering the nutrients needed to train harder and to begin the repair process after a hard workout.

For men, this pump effect is not restricted only to the gym. I have lots of good feedback that a nitric oxide booster such as Arginine can increase the sexual performance in men. Recent studies done by the Department of Urology at Tel Aviv University seem to confirm my findings.

For the best absorption, once again I recommend a powder formula that you can add to your own water. I have been using a product called CardioforLife™. This product contains 5000MG of L-Arginine. This past summer I had an accident and broke my foot. I really did not think this was going to be a big deal other than the inconvenience of having to use crutches for a few months until I found out the fracture caused a blood clot in my calf. This clot in turn then caused me to have a pulmonary embolism, which gave me a ticket to the ER at Wake Medical Hospital and two days of hospital food. Upon release from the hospital I increased my dose of arginine to increase the circulation in my leg. My most recent ultrasound showed no sign of the clot remaining.

Of course in any hospitalization or acute sickness, always let your physician know what supplements you are taking so that there is no drug contraindication or other complications.

5. BCAAS

If you are exercising regularly, including weight training and cardio such as running and cycling then you need to consider supplementing with some Branch Chain Amino Acids. These three aminos; Leucine, Valine and Isoleucine make up about one-third of your muscle protein. When you work out hard, these aminos are the first to go. By supplementing with BCAAs they act as an anti-catabolic agent protecting the muscle you may have spent years developing. They also help you maintain a "positive nitrogen" balance in your body. This is where you want to be for growth and repair.

A recent study of distance runners published in The Journal Sports Medicine and Physical Fitness in the September 2007 issue seems to prove the claim that taking BCAAs before intense exercise can protect the muscle fiber. The researchers were able to measure the actual lactate dehydrogenase (LDH) level, an index of tissue damage in the runners before and after a 25Km run. The researchers were able to conclude that maintaining the blood BCAA level throughout a long distance run contributes to a reduction in the LDH release and, therefore, the effect of BCAA supplementation is suggested to reduce the degree of muscle damage.

One of the best branch chain supplements that I have used is called IBCAAS™ and is an instantized powder form that allows for quick absorption. This supplement can be taken before and during a workout. You can find IBCAAS™ at your local Nutrishop™.

6. GLUTAMINE

To get Bigger, Better, Faster, Stronger you must be able to recover from your intense workouts. As we age our bodies ability to rebuild and recover is reduced. Therefore, we need a little help. That's where the amino acid L-Glutamine comes in.

The Glutamine levels in your body can be reduced by over 50% during your exercise routine. If you stay in a glutamine deficient state your muscles may be depleted of its glutamine stores contributing to further break down of muscle tissue and longer recovery times. Glutamine is also important in maintaining your immune system, intestinal health and wound healing.

Glutamine is typically taken post workout and added to a protein shake. I have used multiple types ranging from tablets to powders. The one I use now is called GLUTACOR™.

7. CREATINE

For a boost in strength, I still have not found a better supplement than good old creatine. When it first came out in the early nineties it quickly became one of the top strength and size-building supplements ever. Then for some reason, it lost some of its popularity. I have recently seen a comeback of sorts with different forms of creatine.

Creatine is a naturally occurring amino acid and can be found in meat and fish. Your body converts creatine into creatine phosphate or phosphocreatine and stores it in muscle tissue to be used for energy requirements. This conversion process in turn readies the creatine phosphate to be converted into ATP, the energy molecule which is used when your muscles contract during exercise. Supplementing with creatine seems to give most users increased strength and in turn quick increases in size and weight. Creatine supplementation affects different people in different ways. If your natural creatine stores are low, you will see dramatic effect. I believe that vegetarians will see some of the best gains using creatine.

There are now multiple forms of creatine with creatine monohydrate being the original form marketed and still the most popular. One downside with the monohydrate form is that some users do experience some gastrointestinal distress on high doses and some bloating with water weight gain. In the late nineties I worked with some of the top sprinters in the NCAA that ran track at Shaw University in Raleigh, NC. They liked the extra power that resulted from creatine use but the weight gain quickly ruled this out for the sprinters. A newer creatine product, Kre-Alkalyn does not appear to cause the water retention and bloating that the monohydrate version of creatine does.

I advise any NCAA athlete to always check with your Sports Medicine Department or Strength and Conditioning coach before consuming any sports nutrition supplements.

There you have it. My top seven picks for nutritional supplements you should consider taking, depending on your goals. To reach those goals, read, and study the rest of this book and come up with a program that works for you.

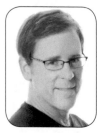

About Philip

Philip Cook, a Certified Personal Trainer, has been involved in the nutrition retail business for the past nineteen years. Philip and his wife, Laura, brought the General Nutrition Center™ franchise chain to the Raleigh, NC market in 1992 and developed six locations. Currently Philip is developing a local presence for another chain based in California, Nutrishop™. Because fitness and nutrition go together, Philip also operates an in-home personal training company, OnSite Training Systems.

To learn more about how nutritional supplements and fitness can enhance your lifestyle, please visit: www.nutrishopusa.com and www.onsitetrainingsystems.com.

CHAPTER 13

Separate From The Pack: From Marine to Strongman

By Tony Montgomery

After serving four years in the Marine Corps and one tour in Iraq, I was finally done. I had served my country valiantly and fought for my freedom. I said to myself, "It's time to let loose." So I did exactly that. Five months and thirty pounds of fat later, I was a mess. I became another statistic, another face in the crowd. I was one of the sixty plus percent of overweight people in this world.

This was something that I thought would never happen to me. I was raised to stand out from the crowd and excel in life. I let myself, my family, and more specifically, my wife and kids down. I took a good, long look in the mirror on August 12, 2008, and knew it was time for a change. On that day, I took my life in my hands and decided to make numerous changes.

The first step was to set a goal and pick a date to do this. I enlisted the help of EliteFTS's own Shelby Starnes and expressed to him my concerns and disappointments. I told him my goal was to get down to single digit body fat within three months. It was a long, grueling process, but I knew it had to be done. I had to take myself out of the majority column and put myself into the minority one. Three months later, I reached my goals. Man, did it empower me to achieve more!

Still, after all this, there was something inside me that said do more, be the best. I decided again that this wasn't good enough for me. I needed something bigger, something more fulfilling. So I set my sights on a Strongman contest sometime in July of 2009. This gave me eight months to transform myself into a Strongman competitor. I knew this would give me enough time to prepare mentally and physically. I set up my template to focus on my weak points while continuing to improve my strong ones.

My template was pretty basic because I didn't know what to expect at a competition.

1. WEEKS 1-4: BASE BUILDING PHASE

Monday

Max effort overhead press	5RM	
Heavy triceps	3–5 sets	6–10 reps
Back	3–5 sets	10–15 reps
Triceps finisher	3 sets	25–50 reps
Circuit abs	3 sets	10–15 reps

Tuesday

Max effort deadlifts	5 RM	
Squat variation	5–7 sets	6–10 reps
Grip	5 sets of random exercises	
Traps	5 sets	10–20 reps

Wednesday

Off

Thursday

Upper body plyometrics	10 sets	3 reps
Back	4–6 sets	3–10 reps
Triceps	3–4 sets	8–12 reps
Biceps	3–4 sets	8–12 reps
Heavy abs	5 sets	8–10 reps

Friday

Off

Saturday

Strongman training
(All I had for equipment was a 700-lb tire Farmer's walk and a sled. I just did medleys.)

Sunday

Off

2. WEEKS 5-10: STRENGTH BUILDING PHASE

Monday

Max effort overhead press	3RM	
Heavy triceps	3–5 sets	6–8 reps
Back	3–5 sets	10–15 reps
Triceps finisher	3 sets	25–50 reps
Circuit abs	3 sets	10–15 reps

Tuesday

Max effort deadlifts	3 RM	
Squat variation	5 sets	5 reps
Grip	5 sets of random exercises	
Traps	5 sets	10–20 reps

Wednesday

Off

Thursday

Upper body plyometrics	10 sets	3 reps
Back	4–6 sets	3–10 reps
Triceps	3–4 sets	8–12 reps
Biceps	3–4 sets	8–12 reps
Heavy abs	5 sets	8–10 reps

Friday

Off

Saturday

Strongman training

Tire Flips	3x5
50' Farmer Walks- (Heavy)	4 Sets
Sled Pulls	4x50'
Weighted Abs	3x8

Sunday

Off

3. WEEKS 11-15: PEAK POWER PHASE

Monday

Max effort overhead press	1RM	
Heavy triceps	3 sets	5 reps
Back	3–5 sets	10–15 reps
Triceps finisher	3 sets	25–50 reps
Circuit abs	3 sets	10–15 reps

Tuesday

Max effort deadlifts	1 RM	
Squat variation	5 sets	5 reps
Grip	5 sets of random exercises	
Traps	5 sets	10–20 reps

Wednesday

Off

Thursday

Upper body plyometrics	10 sets	3 reps
Back	4–6 sets	3–10 reps
Triceps	3–4 sets	8–12 reps
Biceps	3–4 sets	8–12 reps
Heavy abs	5 sets	8–10 reps

Friday

Off

Saturday

Strongman training

Tire Flips	3x8
50' Farmer Walks- (Speed)	4 Sets
Sled Pulls	4x50'
Weighted Abs	3x8

Sunday

Off

4. SHOW WEEK: DELOAD PHASE

Monday

Overhead Press Technique   5x5 50% of 1 Rep Max

Heavy triceps 3 sets 5 reps

Back 2 sets 10–15 reps

Circuit abs 3 sets 10–15 reps

Tuesday

Off

Wednesday

Deadlifts 5x5 50% of 1 Rep Max

Squats 3x5 Light Weight

100 Band Leg Curls

Thursday

Cardio

Friday

Off

Saturday

Strongman Show

I continued to do carb rotation and managed the micros and macros myself. On training days, I consumed a healthy 3600 calories, and on the low days, I consumed 2800 calories. I monitored my weight and made adjustments as I continued to progress. I wasn't worried about putting on 30 lbs of muscle and increasing my deadlift by 100 lbs. That is impossible to do in the short amount of time provided to obtain my goal. I knew if I stuck to my plan and made small improvements I would be fine.

Day in and day out, I was in a zone. All I could focus on was getting in the gym, setting PRs, and crushing the competition. Slowly but surely I was putting on some good size and strength. I couldn't be deterred from my goal, and I wouldn't let anything or anyone get in my way. Finals week in school wasn't a problem. Neighbors complained about the noise, but I didn't care. They were the statistic that I once was and would never be again.

I was obsessed with being the best. I read any and all books related to strength and performance to hone my skills. I had to learn from the best so I took a trip up to New Jersey to train at DeFranco's. I was there for one week learning from the best and training with his NFL crew. That was an experience that will affect the way I do things for the rest of my life. I loved the feeling of being a rare breed, and I wanted more. I continued to set goals and plan my life around the steel. I opened my own gym and continued working on my degree in exercise science all while pounding the weights to achieve my goal.

The day finally came—July 18, 2009, the 3rd Annual SW Florida Strongman Show. I competed in the novice division with ten other Strongmen. I knew I had my work cut out for me. I was undersized in an open weight class, and these guys were on the same path that I was.

First up was the log press—215 for reps in 60 seconds. I pushed out 12 reps and thought maybe I should have tried this before the contest. The second event was the axle deadlift—405 lbs for reps in 60 seconds. I knew this would be my event. I blasted out

13 reps and then my grip gave out. The third event was an 18-lb crucifix hold in each hand. I held it for one minute and seven seconds. Going into the atlas stones, I was in second place and had to set the time to beat. Just before the judge said go, all I could think about was becoming one of the elite and separating myself from the pack.

The first stone was 200 lbs and it went up like a pillow while the second, third, fourth, and fifth did the same. This was the first time I had ever touched stones, and I lifted 200, 220, 240, 260, and 280 lbs like they were my 33-lb, three-year-old daughter. I finished in 15 seconds and waited patiently as the guy in first place went. He struggled with them, and I knew that right then and there it was mine for the taking. It was time to fulfill the life I was born to live. I was separating myself from society, from the pack. The scores were in. As they called out my name and everybody cheered for me—the guy who took first place—I knew my life would never be the same.

I was amazed at the feeling I got when they called my name. That was the validation I needed. That was the separation I desired. That fed me for about two minutes and then I wanted more. Now, I'm on a journey to turn professional, and I won't stop until I get it.

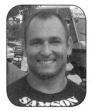

About Tony

Tony Montgomery is training to become a professional strongman and a leader in the strength and conditioning industry. After honorably serving four years in the Marines, he is currently pursuing a degree in exercise science from FAU. He specializes in training athletes of any kind to reach their peak performance. He trains a wide variety of clients from triathletes to football players and everything in between.

CHAPTER 14

A Distinct Physique

By Juan Medrano

My fitness journey takes me back to my younger days when I was 18 years old at a small community gym in the city I lived in. It was the end of my grade 12 year and I was performing what I thought were "great" squats on a smith machine, when all of a sudden I felt a pinch on my lower back. I thought I knew everything about life and working out back then, being a solid 18 years of intimidation, standing at a colossal 5' 6" and weighing 135 pounds soaking wet. I continued to squat and added another 45 pound plate per side bringing my total weight to about 250 pounds. As I proceeded to squat I must have had the most excruciating, painful expression in my face as I was trying to come back up from the squat motion, an older gentleman a couple of machines down from me quickly ran to my aid to help me up, and re-rack the weight. One thing led to another and I found myself in a chiropractors' office hardly being able to walk with my lower back popped out of place. As a result of this, I had the rude awakening that in order for me to continue to work out and stay healthy, I needed to gain accurate knowledge when it came to the science of building a lean and strong physique with no injuries. Years later, through personal experiences, guidance and training from mentors, experiences from working in corporate facilities, and today training clients in my own fitness studio, I have found there is a distinct recipe for getting into the best shape of your life.

There are three training methods that absolutely have to be part of your fitness regimen if your intentions are to lose fat and build lean muscle in a healthy, natural, and sustainable way. These methods will improve co-ordination, posture, core strength, and help you feel and look healthy and young for years to come.

THE THREE GOLDEN TRAINING METHODS TO YOUR BEST BODY

1. The first of the three training methods is called compound movements. These are multi-joint movements for building several muscles or muscle groups all at one time. For example, a chest press exercise engages muscles in the pectorals, deltoids, and triceps all at once. Compound movements are very impor-tant in your fitness routine because they improve joint stability and muscle balance. Also, since you are firing multiple muscle groups at once, you are able to get a full body workout in a shorter duration. Lastly, you are able to lift more weight over time due to less muscle fatigue.

2. Our second method is isolation training. This consists of using machines to increase muscle in size and trength due to fatigu-ing of individual muscles. A great example would be leg ex-tensions, which work only the muscles in the thigh. However, isolation movements may cause stiffness throughout the body or create muscle imbalances if performed incorrectly. There-fore, it is extremely critical to perform isolation movements with great attention to posture and form. Personally, I like to perform isolation exercises immediately followed by an aero-bic activity such as rope skipping or kettle bell swings with my clients, giving them the lean, sculpted muscles they are look-ing for. Isolation training is usually preferred by medical pro-fessionals to correct specific muscles injuries, whether due to muscle weakness, illness, medical procedures or certain medical conditions.

3. Last but not least, we have integrated our functional training. These exercises are related to function in everyday life. Func-tional training helps increase balance, coordination, explosive-ness and strength – due to perfect harmony of muscles working

together as a unit. For example, a push up works the arms, chest, back and shoulder muscles all at once, while engaging the rest of the muscles in the body for stabilization. As a result, these exercises involve many areas and muscle groups all at once to create a full body workout. Functional training is an important component of any fitness routine as it recruits and strengthens muscles that often may be missed in compound and isolation movements.

Each of these three methods used alone will get you results over time. However, if you are truly looking to build a physique that will leave you lighter, stronger, healthier, and feeling better than ever before, you must incorporate a combination of compound movements, isolation training, and functional exercises.

APPLYING THESE THREE METHODS

So, I've touched on the three training methods that are going to get you in great shape. But what does this all mean and how are you going to apply it? Below, I am going to outline a sample exercise routine that would incorporate these three methods to get you optimum results.

Keep in mind that this is going to take commitment on your part. Everything good is worth working for, so if you've been brainwashed by the latest infomercials about the next quick fix...then you're in the wrong place. And if you're reading for the sole purpose of finding a quick solution that's easy... with no investment of time, will, or money on your part... then I suggest you stop reading. If, however, you're finally ready for real talk, and sincere information about how you can transform your body and life in a dramatic way, then I invite you to keep reading, focus, and doggy ear this chapter so you can come back often when you're looking for answers.

While I am not currently writing this chapter on nutrition, I will not go into depth on the topic, however proper nutrition and training must go hand in hand to achieve maximum results. Registered nutritional professionals in your community can assist you with proper nutritional planning to ensure that you will be getting the most out of your exercise program.

Make sure to always consult with your family physician before starting any fitness program.

Let's begin...

Always start with a 5-10 minute warm up and stretch before any type of training, then exit with a cool down when finished. These fundamentals are often overlooked and yet are key elements to any training regimen. The main objective of a basic warm up is to prevent injuries such as muscle pulls or joint injuries. By properly warming up and stretching, you're lubricating all areas of the body by increasing blood and oxygen throughout it. During my routines, I like to continuously stretch after each set because it allows my muscles to relax, and as a result I'm able to comfortably increase my weight little by little, so I can get better gains in time while staying injury free.

The below routine consists of three 35-minutes sessions of strength training, and two 30- minute sessions, of cardiovascular activity for a total of five sessions in a week. It does not matter whether you decide to make your strength training Monday/Wednesday/Friday or Tuesday/Thursday/Saturday as long as you're consistently weight training three days a week. Your warm up will consist of a 5-10 minute power walk, a light jog, running on the spot, rope skipping, high knees, or butt kicks, immediately followed by shoulder and back stretches, calves and ankle stretches, chest stretches, quads and hamstrings stretches, along with wrists and forearms stretches.

WEEK 1- COMPOUND & ISOLATION WEEK

Day 1: Legs

Barbell squats. Perform 3-4 sets for 12 reps. Rest for 45-60 seconds after each set.

Superset (back-to-back) leg press and stationary alternating lunges with no weights. Performing lunges with no weights will keep the knees safe and injury free. This allows you focus that extra bit on correct form as the legs will start to get tired while continuing your routine. Perform 3-4 sets for 12 reps and rest for 45-60 seconds.

Superset leg extensions and lying down leg curls for 3-4 sets for 12 reps. Rest for 45-60 seconds.

Day 2: 30 minutes of cardio

Pick 2 cardio activities on your cardio days and perform each activity for 15 minutes, totaling 30 minutes. For instance you could pick skipping and boxing. The trick to this fat burning process is that you will perform each for 30–40 seconds at high intensity, followed by 15–20 seconds of moderate continuous movement at 50% of the original effort. Repeat until 15 minutes are up then move on to second activity for another 15 minutes. Duplicate same method.

Amazing activities such as swimming, rowing, climbing stairs, kettle bell swings and sprinting will get the job done. Remember that the more muscles used, the more calories/energy burned!

Day 3: Chest

Barbell incline chest press (on a 45 degree bench) superset with cable crossovers for 3-4 sets for 12 reps and resting 45-60 seconds after each set. When done, superset dips and dumbbell presses (presses are to be done on a 15-45 degree angle bench). Repeat the same set and repetition principle then rest for 45-60 seconds after each set. When doing dips, I recommend doing quarter dips for the first two weeks so that you allow your muscles and tendons around their interface to slowly adapt. Once two weeks have gone by, slowly make the progress to half dips. When two weeks have passed and dips have gotten easier, move on to three quarter dips until you're comfortable and strong enough to perform full dips. Once you get to full dips, perform one set to start with and as it gets easier with time and you're staying injury free, feel free to add a second set of full dips. The name of the game is proper progression and training smart!

Day 4: Cardio

Pick any 2 activities and perform each for 30–40 seconds at high intensity followed with 15–20 seconds of moderate continuous movement at 50% of the original effort, and repeat until 15 minutes are up. Move on to second activity for 30–40 seconds at high intensity, followed by 15–20 seconds of moderate continuous movement at 50% of the original effort.

Day 5: Back

Deadlifts. Perform 3-4 sets for 15 reps then rest for 45-60 seconds. Superset seated rows and bent over barbell rows for 3-4 sets for 12 reps. Rest for 45-60 seconds. Finish by supersetting pull-ups – assisted pull-ups is a great way to start. Do 3-4 sets for 1-4 reps performed as correctly as possible, with roman chair hyperextension for stabilization of core and lower back muscles. Once pull-ups get a bit easier, pump out 8-12 reps consistently for 4 sets.

WEEK 2: INTEGRATED/FUNCTIONAL WEEK

Day 1: Functional Full Body Exercises

Exercise 1: Stationary wall squats with bicep curl. 4 sets of 20 reps.

Exercise 2: Pull-up burpees. Perform 3 sets of 12-15 reps.

Exercise 3: Dumbbell triceps kickbacks up into shoulder presses.
     Perform 4 sets of 12-15 reps.

Exercise 4: One-handed chest press into crunch on stability ball.
     Perform 4 sets of 12-15 reps.

Day 2: Cardio

Pick any 2 activities and perform each for 30–40 seconds at high intensity followed with 15–20 seconds of moderate continuous movement at

50% of the original effort and repeat until 15 minutes are up. Move on to second activity for 30–40 seconds at high intensity followed by 15–20 seconds of moderate continuous movement at 50% of the original effort.

Day 3: Functional Full Body Exercises

Exercise 1: Standing medicine ball twists. Make sure to hold the med ball palms in and about mid chest height and rotate trunk left and right always keeping your abdominal core tight by breathing out.
Perform 3 sets of 12-15 reps.

Exercise 2: Superman into a full push-up.
Perform 3 sets of 12-15 reps.

Exercise 3: Medicine ball squats with arm extensions. Make sure to hold the med ball into your chest with your palms in and as you sink down into your squat position, make sure your bum and hips are out and all your weight is on your heels.

Extend your med ball as far out without hyper extending or locking your joints while flexing your arms along with your abdominal core. Make sure to bring your med ball back into your chest as you're coming back up. Again, making sure all your weight is on your heels for great stabilization!
Perform 3 sets of 12-15 reps.

Exercise 4: One arm row alternate with one arm shoulder raise.
Perform 3 sets of 12-15 reps.

Day 4: Cardio

Pick any 2 activities and perform each for 30–40 seconds at high intensity followed with 15–20 seconds of moderate continuous movement at 50% of the original effort, and repeat until 15 minutes are up. Move on to second activity for 30–40 seconds at high intensity followed by 15–20 seconds of moderate continuous movement at 50% of the original effort.

Day 5: Functional Full Body Exercises

Exercise 1: Two handed medicine ball diagonal wood chop.
> Perform 3 sets of 12-15 reps.

Exercise 2: Roman chairs on stability ball with a twist.
> Perform 3 sets of 12-15 reps.

Exercise 3: Rotational shoulder presses on stability ball.
> Perform 3 sets of 12-15 reps.

Exercise 4: Lying down hip bridges with hamstrings ball rollouts.
> Perform 3 sets of 12-15 reps.

Rotate these 2 weeks back and forth; always mix up the order of the exercises to continue confusing your muscles. Muscle confusion is very important as it keeps your body guessing and prevents a plateau effect where you can no longer get results. This is the key element to developing your ideal physique.

In summary, when designing a fitness program, it is very important to include compound, isolation, and functional exercises along with a cardiovascular component. It is also very important to consistently alter your exercises and their order to keep your muscles guessing. If you are new to fitness, be conscious of these methods and seek out fitness professionals who will incorporate a mixture of these exercises. With these concepts in mind, and your commitment, you can achieve the lean, toned and healthy physique you have always desired!

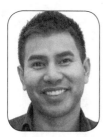

About Juan

Juan Medrano is the owner of Movimento Fitness; a personal and group-training studio located in St. Albert, Alberta, Canada. As a certified personal trainer from the International Sports Science Association with a background in business, Juan makes a name for himself and his studio through dynamic and effective training methods that get results.

Juan's fitness journey began 13 years ago at a small community gym – learning fundamentals in bodybuilding, power lifting and functional exercises from mentors. He has competed in FAME Los Angeles for fitness modeling and has been featured for fitness in local publications and on world FM radio. He continues to gain knowledge from top coaches every year to stay at his best. After working as a trainer in a corporate setting, Juan started Movimento Fitness in April of 2010 and has been going strong ever since, fueled by awesome clients that love the difference they see!

CHAPTER 15

Personality

By Toby Watson

My name is Tobias Kipling Watson (Toby), and I am the owner of CrossFit On the Move – Grant Park and Alpharetta. I want to take a few moments to tell you who I am, how **CrossFit On the Move** came into being, and how fitness is not one-dimensional and is the solution for each of us.

I was born in Albuquerque, New Mexico in October 1980 and grew up in New Mexico as a very active child of doting parents, involved in any and every single sport/sporting activity afforded me. I had a father who would let no impediments stand in the way of my participation. I had a mother who rooted for me no matter what (with and without embarrassment to me). I had an extended family that was embedded in the Land Of Enchantment giving me always a social context of support and identity.

My life since has been one of great mobility, emphasized mostly by my entry into the Army. I have served two tours of duty and left the Army decorated and as Captain. I left overweight, perplexed about endeavor and happiness, and wanting to make a difference. Just prior to separating from the Army I had the opportunity to join the fitness community of CrossFit. I loved the community and the success I obtained within that community, and I opened two CrossFit Affiliates. CrossFit On the Move.

I expected to be moving regularly. On the Move has come to mean adaptable and ready. It has proven a good motif.

LIFESTYLES AND NUTRITION

I created my business and called it CrossFit On the Move because I thought I was going to be in the Army forever and continue to move every 3 years, so I thought it would be a great name. I got out of the Army two years later with two fitness facilities, with a hope that I would be able to continue my growth. Importantly, my own health and well being had been advanced and that is what I want to share with you. Benchmark, identify, and strategize.

Fitness is hard and it is defined by so many things. Fitness doesn't mean you have six- pack abs or can squat a small car. In our community, fitness is constant improvement in many different aspects of life.

Fitness is not limited to but includes all the following:

1) Diet and Nutrition.

2) Physical Fitness (Training).

3) Emotional and Spiritual Fitness.

Fitness begins at the molecular level and that's the Diet. So many people are afraid to address this issue up-front and straightforward. If you walk into any bookstore or online bookstore and look in the diet section, you will find an endless number of "Diet Books." And here is the fact about all of them...THEY ALL WORK FOR SOMEONE!

The way we approach Diets in our community is that all DIETS, capital D, work for the short term, but if you want to have something that works for the long term you need to think of diet, small d, as the way you eat on a regular basis.

Diet with a capital D is a bad word and should not be uttered at all. Diet, lowercase d, is ok. So if you say, "I am on a diet," I will scowl and shake my head. If you say, "My diet consists of these foods," I will smile and silently applaud. Are you able to tell the difference between the two words? It is important that you do, or you will never truly reach your fitness or nutrition goals.

So let's look at the word Diet as in "I am on a Diet!" That has all sorts of negative thoughts and meanings associated with it. You are restricted to what you can and can't eat; you are doing it for a short period of time to fix a problem, and the bottom line is that it is not at all sustainable. So why would you want to be on a Diet? If a diet ends, and you are going to go back to your old habits and gain the weight back, or become inflamed again or whatever the results are after you quit the diet, why do it? Diets also lead people into feeling guilty if you slip up and have a cookie or a beer. You end up feeling guilty for a day or two, and then you starve yourself or end up sneaking food. So diet should become a four-letter word in your house that is not allowed.

Now let's talk about the 'other' diet and what your daily diet consists of. This is a much better relationship with the word diet, because you are using it to mean, "this is the way I eat." Your diet may consist of anything, including whole grains, veggies, ice cream, and beer; but it is what you can sustain, maintain, and eat on a regular basis. You have a good relationship with this word, because it doesn't cause you added stress. You aren't cheating if you eat something like ice cream. Can you tell the difference? What is your relationship with the way you are eating today?

The way we approach Diets in our community is that all DIETS, capital D, work for the short term, but if you want to have something that works for the long term you need to think of diet, small d, as the way you eat on a regular basis.

Diets, capital D, are set up to make you fail. They are quick fixes with lots of restrictions that have a start date and an end date. If there is an end date how can you maintain it? If you are constantly worried about if you cheated or not, you are adding stress to your life – which works against achieving fitness.

So we take a holistic approach to diet and nutrition. Our approach to diet and nutrition is this...first take the word "Diet" out of your vocabulary and use "diet" instead. That simple thing makes it the way you eat normally and you will still see the results you are looking for.

When you are looking at changing your diet, you must first find out what foods affect you in what ways. So we recommend that you take all the processed foods that are in your daily diet and get rid of them for at least 30 days. So you are in fact on a 30-day DIET, with lots of restrictions. What this allows your body to do is to heal itself and get back to its homeostasis.

Now what do I mean by all the processed foods. I mean if it doesn't have a face or a mom and you can't pick it up and eat it in it's natural state then you shouldn't eat it. Another way to look at it is if it comes in a box it's probably not good for you.

So after you get rid of all these processed foods for 30 days you start to add them in slowly. All people are different and react differently to different foods. So after 30 days, add in some bread...so how do you feel after eating it, while you are eating it, the next day. Take note of that. Then add dairy back in and see how that affects you. The slower you add things back in and take note of them, the better you will understand how each type of processed food makes you feel.

Once you understand what foods make you feel sluggish, sleepy, foggy, tired, bloated, etc., you can adapt your diet from there and make educated decisions on the types of foods you eat and when you eat them. My personal example is this: If I eat a piece of bread right now, I will weigh 5 lbs. heavier tomorrow because of the inflammation and allergy I have to the gluten. If I eat dairy, I get zits.

As you gain a greater understanding of the way food makes your feel and the way it makes your body react, you are more likely to make lifelong sustainable changes. You won't feel guilty when you eat a piece of ice cream cake, because you know that is not something you normally do, because it makes you sleepy and not feel good, but you will enjoy it more, because it isn't part of your regular diet.

Changing your diet is not easy, but if you look at it as more of a lifestyle change, and you understand how much better you can feel and look by eating all natural foods, you stop thinking about it as something you can't do, but you think of it as something you don't want to do.

The goal of any Diet, rather diet, should be to allow you to be the best you, you can be. Fitness and diets shouldn't be about losing weight, gaining weight, etc., ...at least not in the beginning. They should be about making you feel and look like your best you! That is the goal.

After we figure out how food affects you, we can then get much more scientific and Diet to get very specific goals. But if you are looking to feel better, have more energy, perform better in all aspects of your life, you must figure out which foods affect you and how they affect you.

It does take a full 90 days for you to completely change your habits and there will be struggles with it. Most people when they switch to eating all natural foods see dramatic change in their body composition, the amount of energy they have, and how they perform in the gym or on the field.

We run Healthy Eating challenges three times a year where we challenge our clients and members to take a close look at what they are eating and make simple changes and commit to those changes for 6 weeks.

So this is how we suggest that you start:

1. Make sure you are eating a protein at every meal. (We prefer animal proteins, but if you are vegetarian there are several alternatives such as Quinoa and beans.

2. Make sure you have a vegetable or fruit at every meal.

3. Make sure that you have a good fat with every meal. These come from several sources, nuts and seeds, coconut, olives, avocados to name a few.

4. Get the processed foods out...(Breads, cereals, dairy, sodas, and artificial sweeteners.

By getting the processed food out and making sure that you are eating a protein, a carb (in the form of fruits and vegetables) and good fat at every meal, your body will almost immediately respond in a positive way.

The stricter you follow this, the bigger the results. What you put into your body is directly related to what you can get out of your body. If you are feeling tired and sluggish, can't sleep at night, are carrying a little extra weight, a lot of that can be solved by making changes to your diet.

Our six-week healthy-eating challenges create huge success for our clients because they learn how different foods affect them and how much more potential they have if they fuel their bodies correctly.

Some of our recent case Studies:

- Tina M, a 40-year-old female, was our last challenge winner. In six weeks she lost 7% body fat, had a 50 pound increase in her deadlift, and was able to complete the cardiovascular portion of the challenge 7 minutes faster than her first time.

- Chris D, a 34-year-old male, came in second place, losing 5% bodyfat, increased his deadlift by 60 pounds, and increased his cardiovascular portion by 5 minutes.

- Elayne, a 42-year-old female, gained 2 pounds of bodyweight, decreased her body fat by 3%, and increased her deadlift by 45 pounds.

By changing the way they were fueling their bodies they were able to see huge cardiovascular gains, huge strength gains, huge body composition changes no matter whether they were overweight or not, and they were able to do so by cleaning up their diet.

The best part about changing the way you look at food and how it affects your body, is that you can finally get off that diet rollercoaster.

The goal of our Healthy Eating Challenges is to show people that if you are pay attention to how different foods affect your body, you can make better decisions and you won't be part of the Dieting crowd anymore. You will have a consistent diet that allows you to splurge on occasion.

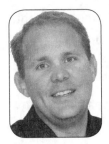

About Toby

Tobias Kipling Watson (Toby) is the Founder of CrossFit On the Move, Grant Park & Alpharetta, GA.

As a former Captain in the Army, Toby discovered Cross-Fit training while in Iraq where he observed special operations forces using CrossFit to stay in shape. While deployed, Toby began utilizing the CrossFit methodology to stay fit and in fighting shape.

After Toby's service in Iraq, he returned to Ft. Benning where he continued to pursue his passion for CrossFit. He constructed a backyard gym, attended his first certification course and began his career in the fitness industry. Eventually Toby purchased a mobile trailer and started training the local community from this trailer. Thus, he created CrossFit On the Move.

In 2009, after completing his service in the Army, Toby opened the first CrossFit On the Move facility in Grant Park. Nine months after opening the Grant Park location, Toby opened a second facility in Alpharetta. With these two gyms, Toby is able to fulfill his vision of creating fitness communities dedicated to helping people achieve their fitness goals and live healthier lifestyles. His commitment to delivering exceptional training, proper nutritional education and information and his functional strength and conditioning programming, have helped drive the growth of both gym locations.

Toby earned a Bachelor of Arts degree in American Studies from the University of Richmond. While in the Army, he was awarded two Bronze Stars and a Meritorious Service Medal. In addition, Toby holds the following certifications:

CrossFit Level	1 CrossFit Kids	OPT Assessment
CrossFit Endurance	CrossFit Nutrition	OPT Program Design
CrossFit Olympic Lifting	CrossFit Kettlebells	OPT Lifestyles

CHAPTER 16

Supercharge Your Health and Fitness with Joint Mobility Training

By Peter Gibbs

Charles came to see me after hip replacement surgery. He was a serious athlete but had suffered with a bad hip for several years prior to surgery. According to his doctor, his new hip was perfect, a total surgical success. According to Stan's physical therapist, he had accomplished his PT goals and could return to his regular activities.

His surgeon told him he should go out and start hitting golf balls again. The problem was, Charles felt like if he tried to swing a golf club he would fall over. He didn't feel stable or balanced when he put weight on his leg. Stairs were a big challenge. He could barely reach his hands to his knees when bent over.

Medically, he was cured, but he still couldn't move the way he wanted to or with any kind of security or balance. After several years of discomfort and a major surgery, he had learned to limit his movement to avoid pain. Although the problem that created the pain and limitation was gone, he was still holding on to movement patterns developed to keep him safe, and avoid feeling pain. These patterns involved limiting the use of muscles that moved his hip and leg. He was 45 and moving like he was 90.

Charles had lots of athletic and training experience and was exercising intensively, working with free weights, doing body-weight exercises, rowing machines and the Stairmaster. Many of the exercises he was doing are considered mobility exercises like pushups, lunges and squats, but he couldn't execute these safely with anything approaching good form. He was working hard, but wasn't getting stronger in ways that would let him do the things he loved, which included bending over to pick up his young daughter and walking his big dog. Charles couldn't move without feeling stiff and old and like he might lose his balance.

In our initial assessment, I watched him walk and asked him to show what movements were hard for him. He did a forward bend barely reaching to his knees. I watched him go up and down a set of stairs several times, struggling on each step.

Things that involved basic movements and balance tasks were compromised for Charles. He was doing high intensity workouts, but his general movement was not improving. He was strong in some ways, but he couldn't activate and control muscles for efficient movement.

I suggested we try something different; Charles was ready to try anything. I had him sit in a chair and gently tilt each ankle, like rolling his ankle to the outside of his foot. I asked him to stand up and hold his left arm out in front of him fully extended, then move his arm in small circles five times in each direction.

After completing these basic mobility drills, I asked him to try a forward bend. His hands reached at least five inches lower with ease. Charles climbed the set of stairs and was amazed with the increased strength and stability in his movement.

Charles was surprised and curious. How could doing such little things make an immediate change in his range of motion and quality of movement? Almost immediately he felt an increased sense of balance, strength and control and within a few weeks Charles was handling the stairs with ease. Bending over to pick up his daughter was a pleasure again instead of a dangerous situation. He returned to playing golf and continues to increase the level of challenge in all of his workouts.

The exercises Charles had been doing to restore his strength and mobility, required too much coordinated body movement. The limitation and compensation he had habitually built into his movement to protect himself were being reinforced by the way he was exercising.

The solution was to start with basic joint mobility training. Initially isolating and improving movements in single joints gave Charles access to more of his movement potential. As a result, he was able take on a progressive challenging program of exercise and increased mobility training and achieve tremendous improvement in his strength, flexibility and movement. Joint mobilizations are part of every workout that Charles does now.

Joint mobility training: it sounds cool and it is. Even better, it is something that anyone can do to become stronger, faster and better coordinated in everyday activities, as well as to achieve high-level performance in sports and dance. Even sitting at a desk is a physical activity with demands on postural muscles: neck, head, arms, wrists, hands and legs.

Why focus on joint mobilization first? It has to do with how we are wired. Our ability to move is controlled by our nervous system. Nerves communicate with our brain super-fast. Joints have lots of nerves that let our brain know where we are in space, how fast we're moving, how much to move and whether or not particular movements are safe. This is called proprioception.

Imagine that you are driving on a foggy road at night. You get cautious, slowing down, spending more time looking to make sure you are staying on the road. You might test your brakes a few times just to be sure. You are on guard for what might go wrong. You probably have tense shoulders and maybe even white knuckles.

Now compare this to driving on a sunny day on a four lane highway with light traffic– you are more at ease and in control. As a result you are comfortable driving faster, maybe even checking out the scenery. On a sunny day, with clear road conditions it is much easier to feel and be safe compared to a foggy road at night. This is what its like in your brain. If it can't predict what will happen when you move your joints, you will slow down, be more cautious, and feel less secure or balanced. When your brain isn't sure how safe it is to move, it will often reduce your range of motion and the amount of strength you can exert. If you have had an injury that limited certain movements, your brain might think it is unsafe to perform and will limit or stop them. Your brain's primary mission is survival and safety. When your brain isn't sure that a movement is safe enough it interprets that movement as dangerous. In Charles case, moving the joints in his leg and hip activated this protection mode. Unfortunately, this can be very limiting. It's even possible for your brain to forget how to move something or create pain to stop you performing movements.

On the other hand, if your brain has good information about what will happen when you move your joints it will let you do much more, becoming stronger, faster and better coordinated. Joint mobilization drills can be thought of as a way to optimize your nervous system for efficient *pain-free* movement.

These mobilization drills have numerous benefits including: increased joint range of motion, improved lubrication of the joints, better body awareness and posture, more connective tissue strength and overall movement skill. Given all of these benefits, joint mobilization training is one of the most important things you can do to get the most out of your health and fitness training.

Ideally, we would all practice moving our joints in all the ways they need to function. Joint mobilization drills start with single joint movements. Over time as you become more proficient, these drills can be done at different speeds, and progressively integrated into more complex movement patterns, to optimize functional movement.

Joint mobilizations are a perfect beginning to a workout. Initially, they should be gentle movements of joints in an easy range of motion. It takes practice and focus. You might be surprised at how uneven your movement can be when you first start, but stick with it. You want to be sure to do good quality repetitions. Most importantly, get some coaching to continually refine your movement and practice.

Seven rules for good joint mobilization:

1. Don't do anything that causes pain.

2. Start and finish every drill with good posture – stand or sit up with your spine long and neutral.

3. Be sure you are balanced – have something to support your balance especially when trying new drills.

4. If it is uncomfortable or not working well, slow down and do smaller movements. There is a tendency to do things "big, fast and hard" in many exercises; that is not the case here.

5. Work toward smooth, fluid, high quality movement. Breath and try to stay as relaxed as you can.

6. Three to eight repetitions – more is not necessarily better.

7. Concentrate. The quality of your attention is directly related to the quality of your movement.

There are precise joint mobilizations for specific issues. Getting some coaching is invaluable, but you can try some basic movements gently, keeping the rules in mind. If you have an injury or medical concerns, check with your doctor before undertaking any activities and remember the first rule: don't do anything that causes pain.

Here are four kinds of joint mobilizations to explore:

1. Ankles:

Sit on something high enough for your feet to be off the floor. Do one ankle at a time. Start off by imagining your foot is in a box. Move your foot tracing the insides of the box: back and forth along the bottom, up and down along the outside, back and forth along the top, and up and down along the inside edge. Do these three or four times. Then try reversing your direction. Once you have a feel for the box shape turn the movement into a circle trying it clockwise and then counter clockwise three to eight times in each direction.

2. Knees:

Remember when you were a little kid sitting on a bench swinging your legs? Even if you don't, you can conjure up an image of it pretty easily. Sit on a high bench or chair and gently swing one leg at a time forward and back like you were a little kid. Then turn that gentle swing into circles. Circle in one direction then the other. Next are pendulum swings, imagine you have one long bone between your knee and heel, swing it back and forth like a pendulum. Remember three to eight repetitions for each movement pattern.

3. Hips:

For many people hip mobility becomes limited, like my client Charles. It can often be accompanied by back, knee and foot pain. There are two options for the basic position, standing or lying. Try this one standing first. Have something to hold on to for balance. While standing with support, extend your right leg just off the floor in front of you, reaching through your heel. Remember good posture. Keep your hips level. Now make small circles with your leg, moving from your hip. If this is difficult or uncomfortable, lie down on your back, extend your leg long by reaching a bit through your heel, lift your leg just up off the mat and make small circles three to eight times in each direction.

4. Shoulders:

Shoulder mobility limitations are a common problem and who doesn't have tension in their shoulders, and neck? Make a <u>relaxed</u> fist, thumb side of hand up; fully extend your arm in front of you. Make smooth slow circles three to eight times in both directions. Try a second position with your arm extended out to your side.

It might seem hard to believe that doing small things can have big results. We all move our joints, but how often do you do it paying attention, being precise and focusing on high quality movement? With proper assessment and coaching you can find joint mobilization drills to supercharge your training and literally change the way you move through life.

For more information and to see videos of joint mobilizations from foot to head go to my website: www.bodymindbalance-ma.com

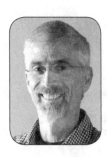

About Peter

Name: Peter Gibbs

City: Worcester, Massachusetts

Company: BodyMind Balance

Website: www.bodymindbalance-ma.com

Work Phone: 508-754-3327

Peter Gibbs, MA, LMFT is the owner of BodyMind Balance, a personal training studio in Worcester Massachusetts. He is a recognized expert in mobility training to reduce pain and the likelihood of injury, while enhancing physical performance at any level.

Peter is a Z-Health® certified Movement Performance and Exercise Therapy Specialist. His background includes bodyweight and suspension training and extensive training in both Stott and Peak styles of Pilates. As a licensed psychotherapist, Peter has expertise in a wide range of motivational techniques. He has practiced and taught meditation and stress management for more than 20 years, and offers a variety of Corporate Wellness programs through BodyMind Balance.

Peter has directed tennis, baseball, soccer and basketball camps and his background in sports performance training is enhanced by years of experience as a tennis professional.

Peter is committed to providing expert coaching to enable anyone, whether a professional athlete or desk athlete, to achieve the highest levels of physical and mental performance.

CHAPTER 17

Going the Distance

By Sarah Graham

How can I be "out of shape"? I am an endurance athlete. As a personal trainer I often have clients and potential clients incredulously ask me this question when I assess their training routine. All too often, endurance runners believe that in order to become better, they need to super-size their training regimen. We know that super-sizing is bad for diet – think restaurant meals and the growth in girth since restaurants have adopted a "more is better" mentality -- and it is equally bad for training. Just as a well-balanced diet with a 'moderation' approach is the golden rule of weight loss or weight maintenance, so too is a well balanced training regimen the key to remaining injury-free and endurance-ready for the endurance athlete.

I know, I know. You're thinking, "Why should I lift weights? I'm a runner." I'm a runner too, as well as a triathlete. Let me tell you why you want to strength train when you're an endurance athlete. There are five primary benefits to strength training that will help you go the distance as an athlete: (1) injury prevention, (2) speed improvement, (3) stress relief, (4) weight loss, and (4) improved VO2 max.

1. INJURY PREVENTION

Nothing kills a good run like an injury that can bench you for not just today's workout, but also possibly for months while you heal. The first thing you want to guard against is over-training. More is not necessarily better. Do you want to train harder or train smarter? I hope you would choose smarter. Strength training will not only allow you to build up your weaker areas, you can also target your weight training to build up important muscle groups that will help to correct your form and technique.

Much of the time, I see people who have come into the gym because they had an injury; most often it's an over-training injury that has forced them to take a hiatus from running. Once we begin stretching and foam rollering their muscles coupled with strength training they see benefits quickly. Many of their injuries could have been prevented with the simple addition of strength training to their fitness regimen.

If you came to the gym for a training session with me, we might begin by working with your lower body and core. In addition to these key areas, all athletes should be working on small stabilizing muscles in relation to their posture, balance and stablization motion for calves, feet, and other small stabilizing muscles in their legs, along with going through complete ROM (range of motion) with their primary movers. A triathlete would want to place an added focus on shoulders, back and chest. A trainer can help you customize a workout for you to incorporate all these elements.

If you are a runner and have not been strength training, there is an increased probability you could have an imbalance of your quadriceps and hamstrings. How does this affect your gait? Imagine your body as one of those old fashioned toys that is a little figurine with rubberbands inside. When you depressed the bottom **button** and release the tension in the bands, the toy falls forward. Your leg muscles function much like the bands in that toy. If the muscles in the front of the leg that control your strength are over-developed, you may have the speed, but the **lack of** muscles **and flexibility** in the back of your body – your hamstrings and back muscles -- will allow you to fall forward just like that toy. Imbalance of strength in the leg can lead to injury or at best cause limited ROM that may cause poor running posture and tight muscles.

If you have over-developed certain muscle groups (like your quadriceps) your body will automatically over-fire these muscles even when attempting to do exercises correctly. You can do even the right exercise incorrectly if you do not compensate for those muscles that over-fire. Strength training will strengthen those weaker muscles, and at the same time allow you to train your muscles to do so with the proper emphasis on the right muscle groups, therefore retraining them to fire properly. This will allow you achieve maximum benefit and maximum power from the training you do.

2. BUILDING MUSCLE IMPROVES SPEED

Contrary to the myth many runners believe that strength training will build bulk and slow them down, strength training will improve your speed by building your "power muscles" – your hamstrings and glutes – while at the same time removing the overuse of your quadriceps. Getting your glutes and hamstrings to fire appropriately will improve your overall speed and efficiency, particularly when running up hills. Doing the neuro-muscular work (that is, mentally connecting to the muscle group that you want to do the motion) in the gym will bring about muscles working in unison. Use your gym workouts as an additional way to train fast twitch muscle fibers without just speed workouts on a track.

I wish I had a dollar for every time I have heard, "I can't do squats" etc. from my athletes! Our natural tendency as humans is to do what comes easily to our bodies. If you "can't" do a certain exercise, maybe you need to find out why.

Your workouts can also be used to improve your core strength and overall upper body, which will increase your speed since even posture and upper body muscles break down at the end of an endurance race. And can we talk about core strength? You would be surprised how many runners, bikers and triathletes I have encountered who possess **poor** core strength. I have them do a push up and their arms can go forever, but their core can't handle one set! Core strength will improve your efficiency of movement. Your core is just that; it's the center of all your movements. A weak core cannot coordinate powerful and efficient movement.

A couple quick things you can do today to improve your core strength are: plank (all different variations like single leg, on stability ball, side plank), reverse plank (on your back, push hips up so just shoulders, head and feet are on floor), mountain climbers, burpees, wood choppers with medicine ball. These are just a few to get you started. Keep in mind changing core exercises in amount of repetitions, sets, and exercises are key to continued progress.

3. GIVE YOURSELF ANOTHER OUTLET FOR STRESS

Come on, I know you love the rush of running! You run for a number of reasons: the endorphin rush, the love of competition, the social interaction you get with other runners, and the overall stress relief of a good run. Think again about the idea that super-sized workouts or too many workouts might be as harmful to your body as a super-sized meal. By using strength training, you can avoid overtraining (even mentally) by harnessing the intensity of weight training as a stress reliever in lieu of running more. Allow your body to recover from endurance fatigue while pushing weight instead of distance. Use your "off season" training as a time to improve your strength instead of harboring the fear of getting "out of shape" or allowing yourself too much time off. You should also utilize lightweight training to speed up your recovery post-race or long run. A simple example of this would be to go through bodyweight exercises such as squat, lunges, side lunges, pushups and calf-raises during your recovery phase. This can help with post-run soreness and allow you to also use them as an opportunity to stretch.

Instead of quickly going through the motions, slow them down and go through each movement to its full ROM (range of motion) holding at any time into a stretch. Follow up with additional stretching, foam rolling, and ice as needed and you will notice how quickly you're feeling fresh and at the same time ensuring you maintain strength and flexibility in your running muscles without the added pounding that may come from a post race run too soon; which brings with it a risk of overtraining from the pounding of running and taxing your sore muscles.

Are you one of those runners who have a tough time with taper because you don't know what you will do with yourself if you can't run? Just think, during "taper" strength training could be a great way to relieve stress without breaking your taper. Injuries come up if you do not allow yourself enough time off between long runs. The best way to recover from the pounding of your runs is to take it out in the gym.

If you don't have much of an off season–you know if you are a race fanatic—it is paramount that you make the best of the time off you do take. Triathletes and iron-man competitors who really have an off season, this is an especially important time for you to hit the gym and work your legs.

4. SHED THOSE EXTRA, UNWANTED POUNDS OF FAT, WHICH MAY BE HOLDING YOU BACK FROM YOUR PR

Believe it or not, some marathon athletes are carrying extra weight. Often times, people train in groups, and the group goes out after a great workout for a bite to eat or celebrate with a victory meal together. Improving your nutrition and adding strength-training to remove just 10-15lbs. can improve your marathon times.

Moving an extra 10-15 pounds the distance of your race will add to your fatigue and recovery time, along with your overall form deteriorating towards the end of your race. Would you run your next race with a lead vest strapped to your body? I bet not. If you are running with extra weight, you are killing your PR just the same.

So how can strength training improve your weight loss? The simple answer is that added muscle will help you burn additional calories during each run or strength training session. Have you considered the toll that those extra pounds are taking on your body? Your knees and connective tissues are overtaxed with every movement when you are overweight. Your run form will not be as efficient if you carry extra weight, and it might keep you from strengthening your core and posture as much as you could.

5. HIGH INTENSITY WEIGHT TRAINING IMPROVES YOUR VO2 MAX

VO2 max is the amount of oxygen your body uses during exercise. This is one area of your fitness routine where less ISN'T more. The higher your VO2 max; the better shape your body is in.

Would you like to double your aerobic capacity in half the time? It's not too good to be true. Instead of running for an hour to increase your VO2 max, specific exercises and intensity a trainer can show you can help you achieve those results faster. Using compound exercises with larger muscle groups and activities such as jump lunges, kettlebell swings, or box jumps is the ultimate in metabolic strength training. Your cardio capacity improves so dramatically that even at your old pace you will be a more efficient machine. If you are really close to your target weight to begin with, your benefits will be seen within as little as two weeks. When you push your muscles with strength demands while at the same time push your heart rate and lung capacity, you are not only improving your efficiency of movement but bringing your body to a whole new level of conditioning that will truly pay off in your race. It's all too easy to get caught up in the hype of the latest trends in runner's magazines. Sometimes these sources can be misleading by only showing you the running side to the successful runner's multi-faceted workout schedule. The fact is there is more to your run than just feet on pavement. That would be a little like assuming the only part of your car you should worry about is the tires!

What other exercise component can you add that will improve your body and your run in five ways? You owe it to yourself to give strength training a try. My suggestions here are some basic things you can do. They are a good starting off point for you to improve your workout; however, form and purpose for what you are trying to achieve are crucial to maximizing your training. A personal trainer can see what you cannot when you are working out, therefore, a trainer can be an invaluable component of your successful training regimen. If you don't currently have a personal fitness trainer, finding one is a good first step on your path for going the distance.

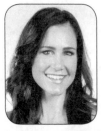

ABOUT SARAH

Sarah Graham is a fitness trainer and businesswoman who specializes in training endurance athletes. She is regularly sought out to speak as an expert and hold workshops for endurance running and triathlon groups on weight training and nutrition for endurance athletes in San Jose, CA. As an athlete herself, she brings her personal experience of knowing what sacrifices, determination, and holistic planning it takes to push towards a PR.

She has studied the physiology of movement and nutrition in college, along with many certifications and continued education courses, teaching methods from traditional, Olympic, functional, rehabilitation, pilates, and endurance running techniques that put her in line with many other top trainers, but what sets her apart is her ability to spot the athlete's weaknesses, find solutions and get results. She asks the questions, "Where is the weak link? What can I do in the gym to build it up and create a more efficient machine?" That is how she looks at the body, as an efficient machine. "I think athletes sometimes underestimate the power and strength that comes from putting their time in at the gym, mainly because they love their sport and want to spend most of their time doing it. I teach them how to increase strength, endurance and improve their movement patterns, which keeps them injury-free and more equipped to reach their goals."

To learn more about how a training program from Sarah Graham Fitness will change the way you race:

Go to: www.sarahgrahamfitness.com or www.personalfitnesssanjose.com
Contact her directly by email at: sarah@sarahgrahamfitness.com
Or by phone (831) 595-1222